STAY YOUNGER,
SMARTER, HEALTHIER

STAY YOUNGER, SMARTER, HEALTHIER

How to Add Ten Good Years to Your Life

Deborah Mitchell

A Lynn Sonberg Book

St. Martin's Paperbacks

Notice: This book is intended as a reference volume only, not as a medical manual. The information given here is designed to help you make informed decisions about your health. It is not intended as a substitute for any treatment that may have been prescribed by your doctor. If you suspect that you have a medical problem, we urge you to seek competent medical help.

Mention of specific companies, organizations, or authorities in this book does not imply endorsement by the author or publisher, nor does mention of specific companies, organizations, or authorities imply that they endorse this book, its author or the publisher.

Internet addresses given in this book were accurate at the time it went to press.

STAY YOUNGER, SMARTER, HEALTHIER

Copyright © 2012 by Lynn Sonberg.

All rights reserved.

For information address St. Martin's Press, 175 Fifth Avenue, New York, NY 10010.

EAN: 978-1-250-00218-1

Printed in the United States of America

St. Martin's Paperbacks edition / October 2012

St. Martin's Paperbacks are published by St. Martin's Press, 175 Fifth Avenue, New York, NY 10010.

10 9 8 7 6 5 4 3 2 1

CONTENTS

INTRODUCTION

A Program to Add Ten Good Years
to Your Life

Mae West once said, "You're never too old to become younger," and there's a lot of truth in those words. Although you cannot turn back the clock and erase years, you can get the most out of the years ahead of you. You *can* stay younger, smarter, and healthier if you embrace and integrate a few life-enhancing, mind-boosting, and spirit-uplifting choices into your everyday life.

What the majority of people want and need is a convenient, doable way to stay as vital, engaged, and healthy as possible without spending a lot of money and seriously disrupting their lives. And you don't need to: all you have to do is make some adjustments—in attitude and in lifestyle—and incorporate them into your life in a way that makes sense and works for you.

I'm not talking about face-lifts or tummy tucks, and I'm not suggesting you check yourself into a rejuvenation clinic or pump yourself up with antiaging hormones. While these options may be somewhat helpful, they are costly, often time-consuming, and don't jibe with most people's budget or lifestyle.

What I *am* talking about is offering you ten doable, effective, and convenient steps—with plenty of options so you can fit them into your own unique way of life. These steps serve one purpose: to help you add ten or more good, healthy, fulfilling years to your life.

What are you waiting for? The best time to do it is *now,* and this book can serve as your guide. Why do you need a guide?

Because there is an enormous amount of information out there about how to fight the aging process. In fact, there is an entire clinical specialty, called antiaging medicine, dedicated to the early detection, prevention, and reversal of age-related disease, using treatments that are based on scientific research conducted by dedicated professionals. And there are also many so-called experts with Web sites and infomercials who claim they have *the* product or *the* treatment or *the* program that will reverse the aging process.

The truth is, there is no one elixir or food or procedure that can add healthy, meaningful years to your life. It is also true that much of the information about how to ward off aging is confusing or contradictory. Some of it sounds too good to be true—and that's because it is. If you're convinced there is a magic pill or drink or injection that will allow you to fight off the aging process without you lifting a finger, then this book is not for you.

If, however, you acknowledge that aging is a process that you can embrace and that you can stay younger, smarter, and healthier if you nurture and support your body/mind/ spirit with positive, easy activities and behaviors, then you've come to the right place.

Stay Younger, Smarter, Healthier is based on a simple premise: if you're willing to take the steps to embrace and challenge aging, then you'll get results. So here's how it goes.

I begin with some background on what aging is—and isn't, and you may be surprised by some of the findings—followed by ten chapters corresponding to a Ten-Step Plan for staying younger, smarter, and healthier. Each chapter/ step covers a major concept necessary to reach your goal: food choices, losing weight, exercise, controlling your health care, keeping your brain young, supplements, social connections, avoiding toxins, stress management, and making your money last.

In addition—and this is the important part—each chapter contains doable, scientifically proven actions you can take to reach your goal. It is up to you to decide which suggestions and options in each chapter will fit into your lifestyle.

For optimal success, you need to adopt at least one suggestion from each chapter, and preferably more. If you share this book with your friends and family—and I hope you do—your choices may be completely different from theirs. But that's great, because your selections should reflect how *you* plan to support and nurture your physical, mental/emotional, and spiritual being as a whole to be younger, smarter, and healthier starting now and for all the extra years you add to your life.

TACKLING AGING: A MATTER OF GENES AND LIFESTYLE

Aging is a fact of life: the body wears down and organs and other body parts become injured, damaged, worn out, and broken down as the years pass. The process of aging occurs at the smallest level—the cellular level—and manifests in bigger ways: sagging skin, reduced eyesight, arthritic joints, graying hair, loss of muscle strength, metabolic changes, and more. Therefore, you need to tackle aging at the cellular level to realize any positive changes on a larger scale.

Genetics certainly plays a significant role in how and why any one person develops certain diseases and medical problems and how that person ages. You can inherit genes that make you more susceptible to develop, say, rheumatoid arthritis or breast cancer, and even if you are more likely to lose your hair, but that's not to say you are guaranteed to develop these conditions. And even if you do, there are certain lifestyle actions you can take to possibly prevent or lessen their impact. No, you cannot change your genes, but you *can* influence how they affect your life, and that influence comes in the form of lifestyle choices.

According to the Centers for Disease Control and Prevention and the National Institutes of Health, the top two causes of death in the United States—heart disease and cancer—account for more than 50 percent of all deaths in the nation. These two categories alone include a great number of different conditions, especially in the cancer category, but even though there are numerous different ailments that make up heart disease and cancer, they have something in common: many of the risk factors for both medical challenges involve lifestyle choices. And that means you can do something about them.

One illustration can be seen in the studies of Seventh-Day Adventists, who limit their use of alcohol and tobacco and follow a mostly plant-based menu (no or limited meat consumption). To this lifestyle they attribute an extra ten years or more of life.

On the other hand, what about genetics? A study released in August 2011 from the Albert Einstein College of Medicine at Yeshiva University reported that among people age 95 and older they found many who had bad health behaviors, including smoking, drinking, lack of exercise, obesity, and a poor diet. So the researchers suggested that based on these findings, genes are mostly responsible for longevity.

But hold on: the researchers also pointed out that genetics is a crap shoot. Scotch and cigarettes may not have killed your aunt Maggie before the age of 102, but you're not your aunt. Your lifestyle choices *do count* when it comes to living a longer, healthier, and happier life, and so you do have a significant role in deciding how long—and how well—you'll live.

Did you know, for example, that exercise appears to have a positive impact on your genes via something called telomeres? (I talk about telomeres throughout the book.) Exercise is just one of the ten lifestyle steps discussed in this book that can help you add years to your life, and telomeres are just one of the factors involved with not only exercise but also other aspects of longevity.

The Mind, Aging, and Longevity

Okay, it's not hard to accept that tangible changes such as an improved diet, regular exercise, and not smoking can ease how rapidly you age and help extend your life, but what about your mind? Can you *think* yourself young?

According to some scientists, if you want to live longer change your attitude. A Mayo Clinic (Rochester) study found that people who had an optimistic attitude decreased their risk of dying early by 50 percent when compared with people who were more pessimistic. Hard to believe? Perhaps you shouldn't be so pessimistic!

According to Dr. Toshihiko Maruta, the study's main investigator, scientists are not certain why personality is a risk factor for poorer health or for dying early. One possibility is that attitude somehow has a negative effect on the immune system. Another is that people who are pessimistic have an increased chance they will experience problems with their physical and emotional health (especially depression) and advancement in their careers.

Being optimistic may not be the only personality trait that can help you live longer. According to psychologist Dr. Howard Friedman, from the University of California at Riverside, mortality and conscientiousness are related. The seventy-year Terman Life-Cycle Study, which looked at personality, social relations, education, physical activity, habits, and cause of death, found that individuals with low adult conscientiousness died at a younger age than did those who were more conscientious. What does this mean? The results suggest that conscientious people may live longer because they are more likely to make concerted, mindful efforts to create physically and emotionally healthful environments in which to live, as they tend to choose more nutritious foods, not smoke, manage their stress levels, avoid toxic substances, remain physically active, and engage in mentally stimulating activities.

Body, mind, and spirit—lifestyle, genetics, consciousness, personality—these and more can have an impact on your health and your ability to live longer, healthier, and smarter. That's why the ten steps in this book address physical, emotional, and spiritual elements in the challenge of aging. I propose you can embrace aging—work with it, not against it, and you'll have a better chance of enjoying a fulfilling, longer life.

STEP 1

Make Age-Defying Food Choices

Would you be willing to change your eating habits today, right now, if you knew the modifications you made could extend your life by ten healthy years or more? Okay, no one can *guarantee* you will live a longer, healthier life if you put down the doughnuts and French fries and go for the fresh fruit and baked potato with fresh herbs. But taking such a step is a terrific start, and one that is supported by lots of research. It's hard to ignore the scores of scientific studies, Internet articles, TV shows, and newspaper reports about the health benefits of a balanced, nutritious diet, even though they do share media time and space with fast-food commercials and stories about people eating deep-fried butter sticks and chocolate bars at the state fair. But deep down, you know the former—and not the latter—is the road to a fuller, healthier life.

If you are serious about wanting to live a longer, more physically and mentally active life, then it is absolutely essential that you provide your body and mind with the best fuel possible. You are probably like most people: you have a pretty good idea of what you *should* be eating, but you could use some encouragement, tips, and guidelines that will make your dietary changes as delicious, convenient, and painless as possible.

You could go to a bookstore or library and peruse the nutrition or diet section. But the sheer volume of options is enough to send anyone running to the nearest fast-food restaurant. That's why this chapter takes a no-nonsense approach and talks about choices that are sensible, doable, convenient, and backed by science.

The age-defying food suggestions in this chapter are ones you can follow for the rest of your life without feeling like you're on a diet, because you won't be: you'll be living with an eating plan that revitalizes you every day. It will also be a program you construct for yourself from the recommendations, so the end result will be Your Plan. If you need to lose weight, then you can combine what you learn here with guidelines from Step 2. If excess weight is not a problem, then you get to skip to Step 3 once you have created your eating plan. Included is a discussion of the pros and cons of calorie restriction, tips on how to eat out sensibly, and some simple, age-defying recipes that you can prepare in ten minutes or less.

SUCCESSFUL AGE-DEFYING EATING PLANS

Of the thousands of eating plans, diet programs, and fad diets out there, only a few have any scientific evidence to back up their claims that they can help you challenge the aging process and the diseases and health conditions typically associated with getting older. I have chosen four approaches that are backed with clinical studies and research: the Okinawa diet, the Mediterranean diet, guidelines from the American Institute for Cancer Research (AICR), and the eating program by Dean Ornish, MD, president of Preventive Medicine Research Institute and author of *Dr. Dean Ornish's Program for Reversing Heart Disease.* Although these age-challenging eating approaches come from different places around the world, they share common features, which will become evident as you read about them, and these common elements make it easy to use them as a basis to create your own personal eating program. Here are the features of the four eating styles.

- The Okinawa diet is based on the food habits of the Okinawan people, who are among the longest-living people in the world. Although lifestyle (including daily exercise), environmental factors, and genetics also play a part in their longevity, diet is a major factor. The diet consists primarily (about 72 percent) of vegetables (lots of dark green vegetables and sweet potatoes), fruits, and whole grains. Seaweed and soy make up about 14 percent, fish about 11 percent, and meat, poultry, and eggs just 3 percent. Green tea and water are the main beverages, and alcohol consumption is moderate (one drink for women, two for men daily). Dairy products are rarely eaten.

• The Mediterranean diet has been widely studied and noted for reducing the risk of overall and cardiovascular death and cancer and cancer death and lower incidences of Alzheimer's disease and Parkinson's disease. Similar to the Okinawa diet, it focuses on vegetables, fruits, and whole grains as the main portion of the diet, but it also includes beans, legumes, nuts, seeds, and olive oil as major items. Fish and seafood are recommended at least twice a week, while poultry, eggs, cheese, and yogurt are recommended in moderate amounts daily to weekly and meat and sweets less often.

• The American Institute for Cancer Research (AICR) advocates a primarily plant-based eating approach and has a program called the New American Plate, which encourages people to look at their plate and change the proportions of food as well as the portions. The goal is to create your plate so that it is composed of two-thirds or more vegetables, fruits, whole grains, and/or beans and one-third or less animal protein. The AICR's expert report, *Food, Nutrition, Physical Activity, and the Prevention of Cancer: A Global Perspective,* found that a primarily plant-based diet may reduce the risk of cancer and other chronic diseases and also help manage weight.

- The eating program proposed by Dean Ornish, MD, is based on a large amount of research indicating that diets high in saturated fat and cholesterol increase the risk of heart disease and that following his eating plan can reverse heart disease. The plan is based on eating 70 to 75 percent of calories as complex carbohydrates, 15 to 20 percent as protein, and 10 percent as fat (primarily polyunsaturated fat). You can indulge in vegetables, fruits, whole grains, and legumes in unlimited amounts, avoiding all meat and dairy products except egg whites, nonfat milk, and nonfat yogurt, strictly limiting plant foods high in fat (e.g., nuts, seeds, avocados, vegetable oils), and consuming salt, sugar, and alcohol in moderation

Before you put together your own age-defying eating plan, here's a quick explanation of the main components of these four eating approaches and why each is important as part of an age-defying plan.

WHAT YOUR BODY NEEDS

Antioxidants and Other Nutrients

Perhaps the most important feature shared by all of the four eating plans is the abundance of foods rich in phytonutrients (nutrients from plants) and antioxidants, including vitamins and minerals. Antioxidants are substances that attack and destroy free radicals, the oxygen molecules that play a key role in the aging process and in the onset of diseases associated with aging, such as heart disease, cancer, osteoporosis, and Alzheimer's disease.

As you get older, your body becomes more susceptible to attack by free radicals, which results in oxidative stress, meaning you have too many free radicals that can damage your cells. To fight those free radicals, you need to maintain a high intake of antioxidants. Antioxidants can help slow aging at the cellular level by helping your cells avoid or minimize damage from free radicals and reduce the effects of aging.

Fruits and vegetables are excellent sources of antioxidants, and the fresher the better. You are encouraged to choose organic produce over conventionally grown, and frozen over canned. Because fruits, vegetables, and whole grains can range quite widely in their antioxidant power level, eat a big variety. (See the "Antioxidant Power Food List" below.)

Antioxidant Power Food List

The antioxidant values of foods are expressed in units called ORACs (Oxygen Radical Absorbance Capacities), which were developed by the National Institute on Aging. The values are based on a 100-gram (3.5-oz.) sample, and the higher the value, the stronger the antioxidant capabilities of the food. However, it is important to remember that the ORAC value is just one measure of a food's value for your health. Foods contain vitamins and minerals besides antioxidants, as well as carbs, protein, and fiber.

Spices are generally exceedingly high in ORAC value. I have only included a few spices, because chances are slim you will consume 3.5 ounces of spices as part of a meal. However, because spices have very potent antioxidant powers, it is a great idea to include them in your eating plan to not only liven up your food but also give a real boost to your fight against free radicals and aging.

Dried oregano: 175,295 (8,347/tsp)	Ground turmeric: 127,068 (6,053/tsp)
Ground cinnamon: 131,420 (6,260/tsp)	Acai berries: 102,700

Unsweetened baking chocolate: 49,944

Black raspberries: 19,220

Pecans: 17,940

Elderberries: 14,697

English walnuts: 13,541

Golden raisins: 10,450

Hazelnuts: 9,645

Blueberries (wild): 9,621

Cranberries: 9,090

Prunes, uncooked: 8,059

Lentils, raw: 7,282

Plums: 6,100

Pomegranates: 4,479

Almonds: 4,454

Strawberries: 4,302

Apple, Granny Smith with skin: 4,275

Cabbage, red boiled: 3,145

Lettuce, red leaf raw: 2,426

Oats, instant dry: 2,308

Black beans, boiled: 2,249

Oat bran: 2,183

Broccoli, boiled: 2,160

Bread, multigrain/whole grain: 1,421

Green tea, brewed: 1,253

And at the lowest end:

Tomatoes: 387

Eggplant, boiled: 245

Zucchini: 180

Watermelon: 142

Cucumber, peeled: 140

Foods That Fight Inflammation

An effective antiaging eating plan includes not only lots of antioxidants but a good amount of anti-inflammatory foods as well. Conveniently, many foods that are high in antioxidants also fight inflammation, especially fruits and vegetables, as well as cold-water fish, which are an excellent source of the healthy fat called omega-3 fatty acids. (See "Fats.")

Inflammation speeds up the aging process and is also a contributing factor in heart disease, autoimmune disorders, cancer, and other serious conditions associated with aging. Therefore, you want to focus on foods that have anti-inflammatory properties rather than those that promote inflammation. Since the four eating plans stress anti-inflammatory foods and recommend you limit or avoid those that can promote inflammation, such as red meat, full-fat dairy, processed foods, and sugars, basing your eating program on this approach will ensure you get plenty of anti-inflammatory foods.

Some of the most potent anti-inflammatory foods are:

- Vegetables in the *Allium* genus: garlic, onions, chives, shallots, and scallions

- Barley

- Beans and lentils

- Nuts and seeds

- Sprouts

- Yogurt and kefir

- Berries

Proteins

Proteins are a macronutrient and the building blocks necessary for the production of cells, organs, muscles, and other tissues. Proteins also have roles as enzymes, hormones, and antibodies.

Your ability to generate new protein and to absorb protein from food may decline as you get older, depending on your health. If you have a chronic disease, such as arthritis or heart disease, then your protein needs may be greater than if you were in better health. However, that does not mean you should arbitrarily increase your protein intake, because excess protein can stress the kidneys and cause a problem with kidney function. Your best bet is to talk to a knowledgeable health-care professional about your specific protein needs based on your health status.

Generally, adults need 0.8 grams of protein per kilogram (2.2 lbs.) of body weight per day to maintain health. That translates into 48 grams of protein daily if you weigh 132 pounds and 60 grams daily if you weigh 165 pounds.

Each of these eating plans focuses on plant protein rather than animal protein, although the latter does play a role. The most common question about plant protein is, "Don't I have to eat certain foods together to make sure I get complete protein?" The answer is no: your body is "smart" enough to combine complementary proteins that you eat within the same day. That means the amino acids in the quinoa you eat for breakfast, the chickpeas in your salad at lunch, and the soy burger at dinner will "get together" and make the protein you need. (See "Sources of Protein.") Animal protein takes a backseat in an age-defying diet, although it is still in the car if you want it to be!

SOURCES OF PROTEIN

- Beans and legumes (e.g., lentils, split peas, pinto beans, kidney beans, black beans, et cetera)

- Soy (e.g., tempeh, tofu, miso, *nattō*)

- Seitan (wheat gluten)

- High-protein grains (e.g., amaranth, quinoa, wheat berries; both amaranth and quinoa are considered complete proteins)

- Fat-free yogurt, fat-free cheese, nonfat milk

- Egg whites

- Chicken and turkey (no skin)

- Cold-water fatty fish

- Lean beef (occasionally)

Carbohydrates

Carbohydrates are another macronutrient and the main source of energy for your body. The digestive system transforms carbohydrates into blood sugar (glucose), which is used by your cells, tissues, and organs. Simple carbohydrates include sugars found naturally in fruits, vegetables, and milk, but sugar is also added to many foods during processing, and this is the type of simple carbohydrate you want to avoid.

All four eating plans focus heavily on complex carbohydrates, which are found in whole grains and whole-grain products, cereals, starchy vegetables, beans, and legumes. Many complex carbohydrates are also excellent sources of fiber, as well as a wide range of phytonutrients, vitamins, and minerals.

Fats

Fats are an often-misunderstood macronutrient, frequently characterized as "bad" when there are actually both healthy and unhealthy fats. Healthy fats include monounsaturated fats, found in foods such as olive oil and avocados, and omega-3 fatty acids, which are found in cold-water fatty fish (e.g., salmon, herring), walnuts, and flaxseed. These healthy fats are the ones you will want to include in your program.

Fats in the unhealthy category are those you want to avoid as much as possible and are found mainly in animal foods such as beef, cheese, and pork, and trans fats, which are synthetic fats found in some processed foods and can be identified on product labels as "hydrogenated oil," "partially hydrogenated oil," and "margarine" and may also be shown under the "Fat" area of the ingredient panel. Both saturated and trans fats are associated with an increased risk of cardiovascular disease and possibly cancer as well, while omega-3 fatty acids and monounsaturated fats are linked with fighting a variety of health concerns, ranging from depression to heart disease, arthritis, and macular degeneration, among others.

Fiber

What role does fiber play in antiaging? Plenty! Maintaining a high-fiber diet helps support brain and bone health, helps reduce the risk of colon cancer, lends a hand in regulating blood pressure, aids in removing cholesterol from the body, and assists in maintaining a healthy weight. Eating foods high in fiber also helps normalize blood glucose levels and bone strength and maintains a healthy digestive tract. Overall, keeping a high level of fiber in your eating plan is a great protective step against many of the health issues that come up as you age. The recommended amount of fiber in your diet is 25 to 30 milligrams daily. (See "High-Fiber Foods" below.)

High-Fiber Foods	Grams
Apple with skin (medium)	5.0
Avocado (1 medium)	11.8
Black beans, cooked (1 cup)	13.9
Bran cereal (1 cup)	19.9
Brown rice, dry (1 cup)	7.9
Kale, cooked (1 cup)	7.2
Kidney beans, cooked (1 cup)	11.6
Lentils, red, cooked (1 cup)	13.6
Lima beans, cooked (1 cup)	8.6
Oats, rolled, dry (1 cup)	12.0
Pasta, whole wheat (1 cup)	6.3
Pear (medium)	5.1
Peas, cooked (1 cup)	8.8
Quinoa, cooked (1 cup)	8.4
Raspberries (1 cup)	6.4
Soybeans, cooked (1 cup)	8.6

YOUR AGE-DEFYING EATING PLAN

Your task is to create your own age-defying eating plan
based on the principles of the four approaches discussed
while incorporating your individual likes and dislikes and
taking into consideration any health conditions discussed
with your health-care provider (e.g., heart disease, diabetes).
When choosing your foods:

- The majority should be vegetables, fruits, whole
  grains, beans, and legumes. Most of these foods
  are high in fiber, complex carbohydrates, and nutrients. Beans and legumes are excellent sources of
  protein, as are some whole grains. (See "Sources of
  Protein.") Picture a plate. about 75 percent of the
  space should be covered with these foods at each
  meal.

- A low to moderate amount of fish, soy, seaweed,
  hormone-free meats and poultry, egg whites, olive
  oil, and nonfat dairy.

- Zero to very low amounts of sugar and alcohol—
  consider them a treat.

- Green tea and purified water freely every day.

So, what's on your age-defying menu? Let's say your current typical day begins with coffee and Danish, followed by
a microwaved processed soup or fast-food burger for lunch
and fried chicken and coleslaw for dinner. A new antiaging
eating plan might look like this (items with asterisks have
recipes that appear at the end of the chapter):

DAY ONE

Breakfast

Quinoa and oatmeal with blueberries*
½ grapefruit
Green tea

Lunch

Spinach salad with tomato, black olives, cucumber, red onion, red
  pepper, chickpeas, and an olive oil and vinegar dressing (you
  can vary the veggies)
Organic whole-grain crackers
Fresh fruit

Dinner

Baked salmon with lemon and cilantro
Baked sweet potato topped with sautéed onions and garlic
Steamed asparagus drizzled with olive oil and slivered almonds
Vegetable juice

DAY TWO

Breakfast

Oatmeal with walnuts and cinnamon
1 cup berries
Green tea

Lunch

Whole-wheat pita stuffed with black bean spread and veggies*
Fresh fruit

Dinner

Tempeh with veggies*
Barley pilaf*
Green salad with tomatoes, grated beets and carrots, red onion,
and cucumber, olive oil and vinegar dressing

DAY THREE

Breakfast

Nonfat yogurt with fruit
½ whole-wheat bagel with honey
Green tea

Lunch

Veggie burger on whole-grain bun, with vegetable topping
Whole fruit (apple or pear with skin)

Dinner

Baked chicken breast seasoned with oregano and turmeric
Twice brown rice*
Spinach salad with orange sections, walnuts, lemon juice,
drizzled olive oil
Vegetable juice

DAY FOUR

Breakfast

Omelet made with egg whites, mushrooms, and bell peppers
Hash-brown potatoes seasoned with turmeric (use spray-on oil in
pan)
Green tea

Lunch

Split pea soup*
Carrot sticks and broccoli florets with salsa
Herbal tea

Dinner

Lentil chili*
Steamed kale or mustard greens with stir-fried onions, garlic, and
    bell pepper
Baked apple with cinnamon

Snack Ideas

Hot-air popped corn with sprayed-on oil and sprinkled with
    garlic powder or chili powder
Organic whole-grain crackers with all-natural nut butter (peanut,
    almond, hazelnut)
Frozen bananas or grapes
Homemade trail mix*
Strawberry freeze*
Green tea smoothie*

WHAT YOU *DON'T* NEED: FOODS THAT PROMOTE AGING

Although it's important to know which foods you should
eat to support your health and longevity, it's also just as
essential to know which ones to avoid. Fortunately, there
are alternatives to each of the types of foods you should
eliminate from your eating plan, and they are offered here
as well.

- **Sugar and sugary foods.** If you want to speed up
  the aging process, bring on the sweets. Sugar and
  refined carbohydrates are not your friends because
  they:

- Cause inflammation, especially of the blood vessels, and inflammation is associated with heart disease
- Are associated with diabetes, insulin resistance, and complications of diabetes
- Interfere with your ability to absorb calcium, which can be detrimental to your bones, heart, and muscles
- Suppress the release of growth hormone, which is necessary for repairing cells and tissues and maintaining brain function, muscle tone, and bone strength

- **Alternatives:** Instead, choose fresh and dried fruits if you have a sweet tooth. The herbal sweetener stevia (no calorie) and small amounts of honey can also be used to sweeten teas, cereals, and other foods.

- **Grilled, fried, or broiled animal products (meats and cheeses).** If a grilled hamburger and fried mozzarella sticks are on your plate, so are AGEs—that's advanced glycation end products. AGEs are a type of toxin absorbed by the body when you eat animal products that are heated at very high temperatures. AGEs are associated with inflammation, insulin resistance, kidney and vascular disease, diabetes, and Alzheimer's disease. Studies show that AGEs play a significant role in age-related inflammation and aging (oxidative stress). **Alternatives:** According to Dr. Helen Vlassara, professor of medicine and geriatrics at Mount Sinai School of Medicine and a researcher who has studied AGEs, you should stew, boil, and steam your food. "Keeping the heat down and maintaining the water content in food reduces AGE levels," she says, and a 50 percent reduction in your intake of AGEs could even extend your life span!

- **Meats and dairy products that contain hormones.** Conventionally raised food animals are treated with hormones (as well as antibiotics and steroids), which end up in the meat, poultry, and dairy foods you eat. **Alternatives:** You can choose hormone-free products or, better yet, switch to plant-based protein sources such as beans, legumes, selected grains, and nuts, all of which are hormone-free.

- **Processed meats.** These are the worst of the worst—processed meats such as sausage, smoked meats, hot dogs, bologna, and salami, all of which often contain cancer-causing nitrites and nitrates. **Alternatives:** If you really crave these foods, try the "faux" meats. Great advances have been made in the taste and texture of processed-type meats made from soy, wheat gluten, and other nonanimal ingredients: soy dogs, soy sausage, and soy deli meats.

- **Conventionally grown produce.** Fruits and vegetables grown using conventional farming methods are regularly treated with herbicides, pesticides, and chemical fertilizers. Even if you wash these produce items well, there is still the risk of exposure to toxins, and there is also some evidence that conventionally grown produce has less nutritional value. **Alternative:** When possible, select organic fruits and vegetables. You can also grow some of your own and use organic, sustainable methods for fertilizing and pest control.

- **Processed foods.** These foods make up the majority of items in many supermarkets. Refined, processed foods contain artificial colorings, flavorings, and preservatives that contribute to free-radical production and aging. Limit your consumption of these foods. **Alternatives:** Choose whole, natural foods whenever possible. Prepare your own "processed"-type foods, such as salad dressings, soups, salsas, sauces, and cereals using natural ingredients.

CALORIE RESTRICTION

"Live long and starve? That's not for me. I like food too much!" That's how one 53-year-old accountant reacted to the idea of calorie restriction. While the idea of strictly limiting your calorie intake for the rest of your life sounds like torture to many people, perhaps it's a bit premature to dismiss it without first looking at its merits.

Calorie restriction (CR), according to the Calorie Restriction Society International, is "the only proven life-extension method known to modern science." It is *not* about starving, nor is it about losing weight, although weight loss is a side effect of calorie restriction. Rather, the goal is to slow aging and extend life span.

And so far, scientific research has demonstrated that calorie-restricted diets do extend life span and improve the health of the many different species that have been tested, including mice, worms, dogs, cows, and monkeys. For example, you may remember hearing about a study in which mice were given a nutritious diet, but some also had their calorie intake cut by 30 to 50 percent. The mice with the restricted-calorie diet lived about 50 percent longer.

Mice studies are okay, but human studies are much more convincing, and an unintended study occurred between 1991 and 1993. That's when eight scientists sealed themselves up in Biosphere 2, an ecological dome in Oracle, Arizona. Soon after they entered the two-year experimental environment, they discovered they would be unable to grow enough food to keep themselves alive. Roy L. Walford, the team's doctor, had been studying calorie restriction for decades, and under his guidance the entire team followed the plan. When the scientists finally left the dome, tests showed improvements in blood cholesterol and blood pressure, an enhanced immune system, and that they were better able to retrieve nutrients from their food as a result of their low-calorie, high-nutrient eating.

Some may consider calorie restriction to be a fad, and although extreme, it does have some scientific evidence to support its claims. The CR Society International is actively pursuing basic research in calorie restriction through long-term human studies, provides information about calorie restriction to the general public and media, and is a contact point for anyone interested in calorie restriction.

But Is a CR Plan for Me?

That's up to you. You should definitely consult a health-care provider who is familiar with the concept and discuss your overall health before taking the plunge. Actually, the recommended way to transition into a CR plan is much more like a very slow river cruise. Dr. Walford, who wrote the book considered to be the CR bible, *Beyond the 120 Year Diet: How to Double Your Vital Years,* recommends taking a minimum of six to nine months, and preferably one to two years, to fully adopt calorie restriction. That said, here are some of the particulars of a CR approach, courtesy of the Calorie Restriction Society International.

Your first question is likely, "What can I eat?" Actually, quite a bit: lots of vegetables, some fruits, low-fat protein (e.g., fish, low-fat dairy, soy and egg whites, turkey, chicken lean beef), and healthy fats (e.g., olive oil, avocado, nuts). The "secret" is to fill up on bulky, nutrient-dense foods that are low in calories—which includes most vegetables and fruits.

When choosing your carbohydrates, select those that are low on the glycemic index. The glycemic index is a measure of how fast a specific food releases sugar into the bloodstream. Most fruits and vegetables are low on the index, while starches such as breads, grains, and dried fruits are high.

Here are some other tips on following a CR program:

- Eat your foods raw or only minimally cooked. This helps ensure you get the most nutrients from your food.

- Chew your food well and eat slowly.

- Know which foods could cause you to "fall off the wagon" and either don't keep them in the house or have only a small amount available, which you use as a treat once a week.

- Plan your meals several days ahead of time so you are not tempted to grab something quick—and high in calories—from the refrigerator or cabinet. It can be helpful to have a list of meal ideas posted on your refrigerator or pantry wall to refer to.

- Try to stick to a daily meal schedule.

How Does Restricting Calories Extend Life and Improve Health?

When you restrict calorie intake, you lower your body fat, and that's a good thing. Too much body fat has been linked to insulin resistance and inflammation, which in turn are associated with a number of ailments and diseases, including diabetes, heart disease, obesity, arthritis, and various cancers.

Your body responds to a reduction in calories by slowing down your metabolism. This is actually a safety and defense mechanism to help prevent your body from breaking down if it's not getting quite enough calories. When your metabolism puts on the brakes, your body not only slows down the rate at which you burn calories; it also affects your cell activity. A slower metabolism causes the body to focus less on reproducing cells and more on fixing cells and tissues. The end result is a slowdown in the aging process.

EATING ALONE

Eating alone can be hazardous to your health, especially if being alone is a new experience for you. If you have lost a partner through death, a breakup, or divorce or you had children living with you and they have left home, you may find yourself eating alone—and poorly. Fast food, microwavable meals, skipped meals—you may feel like it's not worth the effort to prepare something or to take the time to choose healthy foods. But it's more than worth it if you want to stay on track with your nutrition.

If you are in a situation where eating alone is affecting your ability to make good food choices, here are some suggestions:

- Invite a friend to have lunch or dinner with you.

- Have a potluck and invite friends or family.

- Make your meals something special—use candles or treasured dishes or place mats or play favorite music.

- Try a new simple recipe each week.

- Eat meals in different settings: in a park, on your patio, at an outdoor concert, by a stream or lake or a playground where children are playing.

- Look for brown-bag lectures: libraries and community groups sometimes sponsor lunchtime talks where people can bring their own lunch.

- Watch cooking shows on TV or the Internet and get tips on cooking for one.

- Have lunch or dinner with a friend via Skype! Computers now allow us to "be" with others even when we are thousands of miles apart. If you can't share a meal with someone in person, arrange to share a meal while you are on Skype. It's the next best thing to being there.

RECIPES

The following recipes contain ingredients that can help you defy aging: for example, fiber-rich quinoa, oats, lentils, barley, and beans; antioxidant powerhouses such as blueberries, bell peppers, spinach, green tea, tomatoes, and apricots; and plant-based protein, such as tempeh, almonds, and split peas. An added bonus: all the recipes are easy and stress-free!

QUINOA AND OATMEAL WITH BLUEBERRIES

Serves 1

¼ cup water
¼ cup nonfat milk or soy beverage (vanilla is good!)
1 Tbs quinoa
1 ½ Tbs rolled oats
1 Tbs oat bran
Pinch salt
¼ tsp vanilla extract
Blueberries

Combine the water, milk or soy beverage, and quinoa in a saucepan and bring to a rolling boil. Reduce the heat and simmer for 5 minutes. Add the rolled oats, oat bran, and salt, stir, and simmer until thick, about 2–3 minutes. Remove from heat, add the vanilla extract, and serve with blueberries.

LENTIL CHILI

Serves 4

4 cups vegetable broth, low salt
1 small red onion, chopped
1 bell pepper, chopped
3 cloves garlic, chopped
1 cup brown lentils
2 cups chopped tomatoes
2 tsp chili powder
1/8 cup cilantro

Combine all ingredients except the cilantro in a large pot. Bring to a boil, reduce heat, and simmer partially covered for 30 minutes or until the lentils are almost tender. Uncover and cook 5–10 minutes longer. Stir in cilantro and serve.

SPLIT PEA SOUP

Serves 2–3

2 1/2 cups water
1 cup green split peas
1 large onion, chopped
1 large carrot, chopped
2 large cloves garlic, halved
1 cup spinach, chopped
Juice of 1/2 lemon
Black pepper and salt to taste

Combine water, split peas, onion, carrot, and garlic in a large pot. Bring to a boil, reduce heat, add spinach, and simmer for 20 minutes. Remove half the soup from the pot; vigorously stir the soup remaining in the pot with a whisk or hand mixer until it is smooth. Add the saved soup back to the pot, stir in the lemon juice, and season to taste with black pepper and salt.

BARLEY PILAF

Serves 4

1 cup pearl barley
3 cups vegetable broth (low salt)
¼ cup chopped green onion
¼ cup chopped bell pepper
½ cup sliced mushrooms
¼ tsp crushed dried oregano

Bring barley and broth to a boil, reduce heat, cover, and simmer for 30 minutes. Add the onion, pepper, mushrooms, and oregano and continue cooking until barley is tender, about 15 to 20 minutes.

TWICE BROWN RICE

Serves 2

Spray-on oil
½ cup each chopped bell pepper and red onion
1 cup prepared brown rice
⅛ tsp each ground turmeric and oregano

Spray a skillet with the oil and rapidly sauté the bell pepper and onion for 3–4 minutes over medium heat. Remove the vegetables, spray the skillet again, and add the brown rice, seasonings, and vegetables, spreading the mixture out in the bottom of the skillet so it begins to brown slightly. Use a spatula to turn the brown rice several times until it reaches a desirable brown color.

WHOLE-WHEAT PITA STUFFED WITH BLACK BEAN SPREAD AND VEGGIES

Serves 2

Spray-on oil
2 cloves garlic, chopped

1 Tbs minced fresh rosemary
2 cups cooked black beans
Water
2 whole-wheat pitas
Chopped tomatoes, bean sprouts, chopped onion, and chopped
      lettuce

Spray a skillet with oil spray and quickly sauté the garlic and
rosemary. Add the beans and mash them with a large spoon or
fork. You will need to add a small amount of water to make the
beans smooth. Stuff into whole-wheat pitas and add chopped
tomatoes, bean sprouts, chopped onion, and chopped lettuce.

TEMPEH WITH VEGGIES

Serves 2

Spray-on oil
1 package tempeh, cut into blocks
3 cloves garlic
¼ cup vegetable juice
1 cup zucchini, cut into bite-sized chunks
1 cup yellow squash, cut into bite-sized chunks
½ cup red onion
1 cup spinach, chopped

Spray a skillet with oil and add the tempeh and garlic. Stir-
fry until sizzling. Add half of the vegetable juice, cover, and
simmer for a minute. Add the zucchini, yellow squash, onion, and remaining juice. Cover and cook for 2–3 minutes.
Add the spinach, cover again for 1 minute, then serve.

HOMEMADE TRAIL MIX

Makes 3 cups

1 cup diced dried apricots
½ cup dried cranberries

½ cup unsalted dry-roasted almonds
½ cup unsalted dry-roasted sunflower seeds
½ cup unsalted dry-roasted peanuts
1 tsp cinnamon

Place all the ingredients in a big glass jar with a lid; shake well until the cinnamon is distributed.

STRAWBERRY FREEZE

Serves 1

1 cup strawberries cut into quarters
6 oz. nonfat strawberry yogurt
¼ cup freshly squeezed orange juice
1 cup crushed ice

Freeze the strawberries for at least one hour. Add the frozen strawberries, yogurt, and orange juice into a blender and blend until smooth. Add the crushed ice and blend again.

GREEN TEA SMOOTHIE

Serves 1

1 cup strong green tea
½ cup nonfat plain yogurt
½ cup honeydew melon in chunks
Stevia for sweetness, if desired

After making the tea, cool it and pour into an ice cube tray and freeze. After the tea has frozen, put the cubes in a blender with the yogurt and honeydew and blend until smooth. Add more honeydew if you want a thicker smoothie. Add stevia for sweetness, if desired.

STEP 2

Lose Weight to Add Years

Are you carrying some excess weight? If so, you're definitely not alone. Approximately two-thirds of adults in the United States are either overweight or obese, and those extra pounds are doing more than weighing people down: that weight is also cutting into their life span.

Regardless of your age, excess pounds can pose a health risk and contribute to or cause a variety of medical problems, as well as accelerate the aging process. Nature's cruel joke, of course, is that it gets more difficult to lose weight as we get older. That doesn't mean it's too late to drop those extra pounds; in fact, following the other steps in this book can help you in your quest to lose weight. Why? Because as you take the steps necessary to improve your physical, mental, and emotional health and add years to your life your overall attitude will change. You will feel better about yourself and your goals, and when your self-esteem improves so will your motivation to keep improving. And as anyone who has tried to lose weight knows, it can take a great deal of motivation to keep on track.

This chapter provides motivation and helps you "beat" nature to lose those extra pounds using a variety of diet, exercise, and mind/body approaches you can incorporate into your lifestyle. I also explain the science behind the suggested methods.

WHY LOSING WEIGHT IS MORE DIFFICULT
WITH AGE: STILL NO EXCUSE

It's generally known and accepted that it's more difficult to lose weight as you get older. Lots of people blame it on a slowing down of their metabolism and that is partially true, but it's definitely not the whole story. If you want and need to lose weight, then the following explanations for why it's harder to drops pounds as we age should not be viewed as excuses but as knowledge you can use to overcome the challenge and lose those excess pounds so you can live a longer, healthier life.

You are always burning calories, even when you sleep. But beginning around age 40, in order to maintain your weight you actually have to eat about 100 fewer calories per day. That's because your resting metabolic rate begins to change. If you keep eating the same amount of calories per day, you will gain about ten pounds per year. If, however, you reduce your daily intake by 100 calories, you should maintain your weight.

I realize this is an oversimplification, because there are other elements involved, including the amount of exercise you do and health problems you may have, but you can use this 100-calorie-per-day factor as a starting point for weight loss, which is discussed in the next section.

Other factors can complicate the quest to lose weight—or even maintain weight—as you age. Some of those factors have to do with lifestyle: you are busy with work and don't exercise as much as you should, you are invited out to eat with coworkers or friends and family, you have children and you may tend to eat more junk food, you travel and eat poorly on the road, or you may mindlessly eat late at night after a hard day at work. The point is, excess weight doesn't suddenly appear overnight like an unexpected package: it creeps on slowly as you go about your life, and so you need to make small changes in your habits to avoid its insidious advance.

Among women more than men, problems with thyroid

function begin to appear as they age. Since the thyroid is intimately involved with metabolism, and hypothyroidism (low thyroid function, which results in weight gain) is a problem among women, issues with thyroid function can be a challenge (but a solvable one with medication) among women.

Yet another change is in muscle mass, which affects both men and women, although again women are hit harder, because on average they lose muscle mass twice as fast as men. A reduction in muscle mass occurs throughout the body, affecting skeletal muscle, heart muscle, and other muscles that affect organ function. Loss of muscle mass can make a significant difference in the ability to lose and maintain weight. Because muscle is metabolically more active than fat tissue, people who have more muscle burn more calories than those who have more fat. That's why it's so important to preserve muscle as you get older. (See Step 3 on exercise and strength training.)

Then a funny thing happens when you reach a more advanced age, say, around 70 or 80. That's when people tend to slowly lose weight. Although this does not affect everyone who reaches these decades, it is a common trend, and experts believe it is related to hormonal and metabolic changes and even the fact that people modify their dietary habits because they lose their appetite due to health or social reasons.

So those are the main reasons why people tend to gain weight as they age. But what can you do about it?

WHY EXCESS WEIGHT CONTRIBUTES TO AGING

Researchers have found scientific evidence that excess weight can have a negative impact on aging, and it involves a structure in the body called telomeres. In fact, telomeres are one of the "hottest" indicators of aging, so you will be reading a lot more about them throughout this book.

In simple terms, telomeres are sequences of DNA (genetic

code) located at the ends of chromosomes. These telomeres protect genetic information, help cells divide, and are involved in the aging process and how people get cancer. Telomeres are like tiny protective caps that prevent the ends of chromosomes from being damaged and sticking to each other. If either of these unfortunate events happens, genetic information can get mixed up and cause cancer, other diseases, or death.

Every time a cell divides, the telomeres get shorter. When the telomeres become too short, a cell reaches a point when it can't divide anymore and it becomes inactive or dies. This process is associated with aging.

How does this relate to weight? Collaboration between experts from the United States and Britain found that the more people weigh, the older their cells appear under a microscope, and that fat speeds up the aging process. The investigators looked at blood samples from 1,122 women ages 18 to 76, including 119 who were obese. When the researchers examined the telomeres of the participants' white blood cells, they noticed a direct relationship between body weight and the length of the telomeres: lean women had significantly longer telomeres than the heavy women, and obese women (body weight index of 30 or higher) had the shortest telomeres.

In fact, the study's authors concluded that obesity adds nearly nine years to a person's body—that is, an obese individual who is 65 has the body of a 74-year-old person. According to Tim Spector of St. Thomas' Hospital in London, who led the study, "We've known obesity increases your risk of many diseases, and of dying early. What's novel here is that it seems that fat itself actually accelerates the aging process." The investigators also observed that the higher the levels of leptin (a hormone produced by fat cells) found in the blood, the shorter the telomeres.

Since the body is a holistic organism and every factor has either a direct or indirect impact on all other factors, excess weight is just one contributor to the aging process. Weight is also intimately linked to diet, exercise, and lifestyle choices, which also have an effect on aging. That's why it is important to address every step in the quest to live healthier, longer, and not just one. If you could benefit from weight loss, now is the time to do it.

SUCCESSFUL WAYS TO LOSE WEIGHT

If you are looking for a magic weight-loss formula or potion, sorry, there is none. However, now that you know the facts about aging and weight challenges, you can do something about them. Before you begin answering your weight-loss question, talk to your health-care professional about your plan. If you believe you are experiencing some problems with your thyroid, this is the time to bring it up with your doctor. Simple blood tests can be ordered to check thyroid functioning.

Otherwise, let's begin.

Fewer Calories, More Nutrition

First, you will need to eat less calories but not necessarily less food. In fact, if you are smart about taking this step, you may end up eating more food but fewer calories. The eating suggestions offered in Step 1 are an excellent place to start, because they emphasize foods that are high in fiber (which helps satisfy your hunger) and nutrients while providing low to moderate amounts of calories and fat.

Before you can begin to modify your eating habits, it helps to know what you are eating now. Write down everything you eat—all meals, snacks, the cookie you scooped up off the counter on your way out to the store, your grandchild's leftover applesauce—and some notes about when you ate: while watching TV, out with friends, in the car, or with the family. Make sure you include every bit of salad dressing, butter on your toast, oil in cooking, sugar in your coffee—everything.

How is your current way of eating different from the

recommendations in Step 1? Oceans apart? Not too far off? All that matters is that you begin to make changes, gradually and consistently. Here are a few suggestions on how to make modifications.

INSTEAD OF. . . . TRY

- Baked potato with sour cream and butter . . . sweet potato with salsa

- Sugar frosted flakes and milk . . . oatmeal and berries (or plain cornflakes with nonfat vanilla soy beverage)

- Macaroni and cheese . . . whole-grain pasta and marinara sauce

- Cheese omelet . . . egg-white omelet with bell peppers and mushrooms

- Fried fish and French fries . . . poached salmon and baked fries

- Fast-food hamburger . . . veggie burger (no bun) with tomato, lettuce, onion, and salsa

- Fried chicken, mashed potatoes, and gravy . . . baked or broiled chicken, brown rice, and steamed veggies

- Green salad with creamy dressing . . . green salad with drizzled olive oil, vinegar, and herbs

- Beef and cheese burrito . . . stir-fried veggies wrapped in a whole-grain tortilla

- Dish of ice cream . . . smoothie made with fresh fruit and nonfat yogurt

- Potato chips and dip . . . raw veggies and salsa

- Fruit drinks and/or regular sodas . . . green tea, water with lemon

Depending on your current eating habits, you can likely eliminate several hundred calories per day just by changing your use of condiments, dressings, gravies, and sugars. If you need to lose only ten or fifteen pounds, eliminating 300 to 400 calories per day and increasing your exercise (which is discussed next) could help you drop the weight at a rate of about two pounds per month. If you have more weight to lose, you will need to cut back on more calories.

Keep this in mind when you are developing your weight-loss strategy:

- You need to eat at least 100 fewer calories per day beginning around age 40 just to maintain weight. Therefore, to begin losing weight, you will need to eliminate more than 100 calories per day; and

- You need to reduce your calorie intake by 3,500 calories to lose 1 pound. If a 12-ounce can of cola is 150 calories and you now drink 2 per day, you could lose 2 pounds per month if you switched to a no-calorie beverage (once you cut the other one hundred calories per day, that is).

Beware of Beverages

I want to highlight beverages because these are items it is easy to "forget" have calories. Consider the popular latte, which is a combination of coffee, milk (nonfat, regular, soy), and flavorings, including sugar. They can weigh in at 150 to 400 calories or more for just one drink. That's a lot of calories, and with very little nutritional value as well. Nondiet sodas are made with artificial sugars that are considered toxins (see Step 8), and most fruit drinks are full of sugar and few nutrients. Pure water, green tea, and some herbal teas (the latter sometimes have added sugars) are your best bet when it comes to healthy beverages without calories. Homemade vegetable and fruit juices can be nutritious choices when used in place of fruit and vegetable servings, but leave in some of the pulp so you get fiber.

The truth is, many people find that if they make a lifestyle change to a new eating style as explained in Step 1 and expanded on here they lose weight. Because the foods described in Step 1 are an age-defying way to eat, following this plan can add years while you drop pounds. If there is a secret to this way of eating, it's consistency: keep doing it and it will work.

Increase Aerobic Exercise

I know it doesn't seem fair, but as you get older the same exercise you did when you were younger doesn't give you the same results because your metabolism has cranked down. So if you used to walk 1.5 miles a day to maintain your weight, you'll need to increase your efforts. You can do this in several ways: add more time and/or distance to your regular workout, add another day of exercise to your week, and/or make your routines more vigorous.

For example, if you walk 1.5 miles three times a week and take an aerobics class twice a week, you can up your mileage to 2 miles per session or increase your walking to 2 miles twice a week and take aerobics three times a week. Or, if you use a treadmill three times a week, you could increase intensity by adding incline to your workouts instead of walking or jogging on a level surface.

Now may also be the time to add something new as part of your exercise routine.

- Activities such as tai chi, qigong, and yoga are effective stress reducers as well as good forms of exercise that can improve your flexibility, balance, and muscle tone.

- Dance is another activity that is fun as well as physical, and you don't need to be a great dancer or even have a partner to do it. Tap, jazz, modern, ballet, belly, and line dancing can be done solo or in a group. You can practice at home or with others; take lessons in person or from a DVD or the Internet.

- Get physical with Wii. The Nintendo Wii exercise games are definitely not just for kids but great for the young at heart. Options include yoga, strength training, aerobics, and many different sports, including tennis, bowling, baseball, and more. I'm not suggesting you run out and purchase the equipment, but if you already have Wii and aren't utilizing it you may be missing a great opportunity to add exercise, fun, and years to your life. If you are thinking about buying the product, try some of the activities available before purchasing to make sure you like it.

- Consider joining a team or exercise group. You may work for a company that has a bowling, tennis, or baseball team, or there may be one in your neighborhood, at a nearby community center, senior center, school, or church. Some communities have walking or jogging clubs, formal or informal, that meet at parks, shopping malls, or school tracks.

Increase the amount of physical activity in your life in other ways so it becomes a habit and not the exception. For example:

- Use the stairs instead of escalators and elevators when practical.

- Park far enough away from stores and other places you drive to so you have to walk farther (when safe, of course).

- If you take public transportation, get off at the stop before your regular one and walk (again, if safe).

- Stretch and do simple exercises while watching TV.

- Set aside part of your lunch breaks and coffee breaks to walk.

- Rake leaves instead of using a leaf blower.

- Wash your car instead of taking it to a car wash.

- Offer to walk your neighbor's dog.

- If there are any services within walking distance of your house or work, walk to them.

See more about aerobic exercise in Step 3.

Increase Your Muscle Strength

Muscle cells burn more calories than fat cells, both while you are active and even during resting times. First, however, you need to build some muscle by calling into service all your major muscle groups. Because building muscle strength is a component of Step 3 on exercise, I won't go into detail here: you can get the particulars on how to increase muscle strength in the next chapter.

I do want to stress, however, that increasing your muscle strength works in two main ways for weight loss. One, you burn calories while you are performing the training sessions. You don't need to do hours and hours of strength training, just about fifteen to twenty minutes three times per week. The weights you choose should be heavy enough to challenge you but not so heavy they can harm you. Many women who first start with strength training, for example, use 1- or 2-pound hand weights to do their arm exercises.

Two, strength training is a gift that keeps on giving: the muscle tissue you develop will burn up more calories than the fat tissue it replaced. For best fat-burning results, you should do exercises in each of the major muscle groups, which includes the neck, trapezoids, shoulders, lats, biceps, chest, triceps, lower back, thighs, butt, and abdominals. I know this sounds like a lot of work, but you won't exercise every muscle group in each session. You'll see what I mean in Step 3.

EXTRA TIPS TO HELP YOU LOSE WEIGHT

- **Get enough sleep.** Did you know that insufficient sleep can contribute to weight gain? There are several reasons this occurs. One is a tendency to reach for comfort, pick-me-up foods when you are feeling sleepy. Low on energy? How about a candy bar or a few cookies? It's easy to do without even thinking about it. Feeling tired or sleepy is also a reason people give for skipping their daily exercise or picking up fast food instead of cooking something nutritious. One more side effect of not enough sleep—your metabolism slows down, so you burn fewer calories.

- **Don't let yourself get too hungry.** When you do, it's much too easy to overeat at the next meal.

- **Drink water or green tea.** When you keep yourself properly hydrated, you can more easily fight off the feelings of hunger and eliminate toxins from your body.

- **Seek support.** Following a weight-loss program is a challenge, so why go it alone? Get support and encouragement from every possible source: friends, family, motivational tapes, weight-loss Web sites and podcasts, commercial weight-loss programs, a trusted health-care professional, forums, chat rooms, books.

- **Consider natural supplements.** With the blessings of your health-care professional, you might consider using a natural remedy that may provide some assistance with your weight-loss efforts. Although manufacturers of dozens of herbal remedies claim their products can help with weight loss, very few have viable scientific evidence to back them up. Those that look the most promising are conjugated linoleic acid (CLA), chitosan, irvingia gabonensis, and pyruvate.

Eat Out Without Overdoing It

Your best friend wants to meet for dinner, you have a big company party to attend, or your family is having a get-together and it involves lots of food. What's the first thing you do—skip breakfast and lunch, right? Wrong! This is the classic mistake people make when they want to "make sure" they don't eat too many calories at a party or special dinner. Unfortunately, because they are so hungry when they finally get to dinner they *do* eat too much.

If you want to eat out without overdoing it and consuming too many calories, there are a few general tips you can follow. Remember, it is very possible to eat well, enjoy your family and friends, and still lose weight. Here's how:

- **Don't show up starving.** Instead, eat a light lunch or at least a light snack to keep your hunger under control. Meals consisting of protein and complex carbs, such as a mixed-green salad with some garbanzo beans or walnuts, a low-fat yogurt with fresh fruit, or a smoothie, are excellent ways to stave off the superhungries.

- **Ignore the bread and cracker basket.** Ditto for the chips and dips. Unless you are someone who can eat just one small piece of bread without smothering it in butter or just a few chips, then it is best to pretend these tempting tidbits are not on the table.

- **Go easy on the alcohol.** For best health, women should have no more than 1 and men no more than 2 drinks per day. If you want to be social but avoid the extra empty calories, ask for sparkling water with lime or a dash of cranberry juice.

- **Watch your portions.** If you think a menu entrée will give you more food than you should eat, you have several choices: you can eat part of it and take the rest home, you can share the entrée with someone else, or you can choose to have two appetizers or sides (veggies) instead of an entrée.

- **Start with soup.** A low-calorie hot soup (e.g., miso, vegetable) can cut your hunger and help you from overeating. Skip the creamy soups and bisques and hold the crackers. Often, soup and a side dish is an adequate meal.

- **Ask questions about the menu items.** Just because a menu item is advertised as "light" or "low
calorie" or "healthy" doesn't mean it really is. Ask
about the ingredients and how an item is made or
served. If the answer is fried, with butter or gravy,
breaded, or cooked in oil, ask if the item can be
prepared differently—steamed, without the fats or
oils, et cetera. Choose lean protein (e.g., broiled
chicken or seafood), whole grains (e.g., brown rice,
whole-wheat pasta), and steamed vegetables.

- **Be salad savvy.** If the salad comes with the meal
or can be ordered separately, ask for the dressing
(low calorie) on the side and limit or skip the bacon
bits, cheese, croutons, and crispy noodles. If you
are at a salad bar, the same warnings apply, plus
choose a wide assortment of greens and veggies.
If the salad is your meal, be sure to add protein
(beans, edamame, nuts).

- **Avoid all-you-can-eat establishments.** These are
a land mine.

- **Keep a beverage in your hand.** If you are at a
party or work-related event, keep a non- or low-
calorie beverage in your hand—it gives you something to sip and helps you avoid picking up food.

STEP 3

Exercise for Fun and Energy

The human body was made to move. Physical activity benefits every fiber of your being, regardless of your age. You don't have to be like the fitness guru Jack LaLanne, who continued his daily two-hour exercise routine until the day before he died at age 96 of respiratory failure, or fitness icon Jane Fonda, who was still releasing exercise videos at age 72.

But to add productive years to your life, it is necessary to embrace physical activity as part of your daily routine. Exercise has a positive impact on your blood chemistry, blood vessels, heart, bones, and muscles—your entire body and even your mood. Regular exercise changes your blood chemistry, and balanced blood chemistry is critical because your blood impacts the integrity of your blood vessels.

If you want to exercise to help stay smarter, younger, and healthier, you need to exercise smart—with your head as well as your body. How you choose to incorporate exercise into your lifestyle will differ from how anyone else does it, because your plan will depend on your age, current health status, physical-activity likes and dislikes, family and work schedule, even where you live.

HOW EXERCISE FIGHTS AGING

Although your body and all its components undergo a natural aging process, physical activity can apply the brakes to some of the wear, tear, and deterioration and, as a result, add years and vitality to your life. Research shows that you can begin reversing the aging process regardless of your age if you exercise—even if you've been a couch potato.

Here are some of the main benefits you will get when you recruit physical exercise to fight aging:

- **Help in preventing obesity and weight gain.** As mentioned in Step 2, it becomes more difficult to lose weight as you age, but adding exercise to your lifestyle or stepping up your current physical activity can help prevent weight gain or be your weight maintenance friend.

- **Maintenance of cardiovascular health.** It's not just your joints that may get a bit stiff as you age; your arteries become stiffer, too, as the chemical composition of the artery walls changes. This change makes it more difficult for blood to flow efficiently, causes changes in blood pressure, and thus stresses the heart. You can help slow or reverse this damage by engaging in regular aerobic exercise.

- **Promotion of muscle strength.** Your body loses muscle mass at a rate of about 1 percent a year beginning in middle age. You can either let it happen or engage in muscle-strengthening activities and offset this muscle loss. Exercising for muscle strength is critical as you age, especially your leg muscles, because you want to maintain good balance and avoid falls, which often result in fractures.

- **Support of bone health.** Bone may look like a hard, lifeless object, but it is living tissue, and it responds to exercise by getting stronger. For most people, bone mass reaches its peak during their twenties and after that it begins to decline. Weight-bearing exercise, such as walking, jogging, tennis, dancing, and weight training, all force you to work against gravity, which helps build bone. Another way exercise supports bone health is that it allows you to maintain muscle strength, balance, and co-ordination, which then helps prevent falls and fractures. Given that osteoporosis is such a common problem among older adults, it pays to exercise to help prevent this bone-thinning disease.

- **Control of inflammation.** "Inflammation" is one of the major buzzwords when it comes to disease and aging, mostly because the process of inflammation not only can worsen with age; it also is involved in a multitude of ailments and diseases—ranging from atherosclerosis to cancer and obesity—that can shorten your life unless you take action. Briefly, inflammation is the body's response to injury or damage to tissues and that response involves swelling, pain, and loss of function. Inflammation can occur anywhere in the body, including blood vessels, muscles, and the tissues of the internal organs. Exercise is a major action you can take to reduce inflammation. In a study that evaluated data from the Health, Aging, and Body Composition Study involving 3,076 adults ages 70 to 79, for example, researchers found that inflammatory markers like C-reactive protein were lower in subjects who exercised more.

- **Reduction of depression.** When you exercise, you trigger the release of feel-good chemicals called endorphins. These chemicals interact with the receptors in your brain that reduce how you perceive pain, work to elevate your mood, and provide a sedative effect as well. If you have ever participated in a workout that left you feeling euphoric, you have experienced what some call a runner's high, although you don't have to be a runner to enjoy this feeling. The positive impact of physical exercise is so well recognized that many health-care providers recommend exercise as part of a treatment plan for their patients who are depressed.

- **Improvement of blood chemistry.** There's a new field called metabolomics, which is the study of chemicals in the blood, and some researchers from Harvard—Robert Gerszten and Greg Lewis—are making headway in several areas, including the effects of exercise on the blood. In 2011 they reported they had found significant changes took place in the blood after just a short spurt of exercise among healthy volunteers, who ran for about ten minutes on a treadmill. Blood samples were taken before exercise, as the test ended, and one hour later. After just ten minutes, the level of glycerol, a marker of the body's ability to burn fat, was up, as was glucose-6-phosphate, an indicator of the use of energy stored in the muscles and liver. Several other substances had increased as well, and all this is an indication that the body revs up how it deals with potentially harmful by-products of free radicals fairly quickly. Thus exercise quickly improves blood chemistry.

- **Boosting of the immune system.** Experts have come up with several theories about why exercise improves immunity. The actual reason may be one or more of these ideas, and likely others as well:
  - Exercise causes your body temperature to rise, creating a type of "fever." Since your body raises your body temperature when you have an

infection as a way to fight and kill the pathogens, exercise could be a way your body naturally fights off infection.

- Exercise increases oxygen in the bloodstream, while oxygen deficiency leads to a decline in immune function. Immune system cells such as killer and natural killer T cells need oxygen to fight viruses and tumors.

- Exercise deepens breathing, and this in turn stimulates the lymph system. Movement also stimulates lymph circulation. An improvement in lymph system functioning means more immune cells can be transported to areas where they are needed to defend the body.

- Exercise reduces stress and tension, both of which can interfere with your immune system's ability to function at its best.

- **Removal of toxins that contribute to aging.** Physical activity increases the speed at which your body can eliminate waste and toxins through your breath (faster breathing rate) and sweat.

- **Reduction of diabetes risk.** Aging has a negative effect on your body's ability to control blood sugar levels, which means you are more likely to develop diabetes. To this fact add the tendency to gain weight with increasing age and you have a recipe for diabetes. Aerobic exercise forces the muscles to take up sugar from the bloodstream and use it for energy, which keeps blood sugar levels down. Thus a regular, steady exercise program can help reduce your risk of developing type 2 diabetes.

- **Maintenance of healthy telomeres.** One of the "hottest" indicators of aging is telomeres, which are sequences of DNA (genetic code) located at the ends of chromosomes. These telomeres protect genetic information, help cells divide, and are involved in the aging process and how people get cancer. Telomeres are like tiny protective caps that prevent the ends of chromosomes from being damaged and sticking to each other. When this happens, genetic information can get mixed up and cause cancer, other diseases, and death. Every time a cell divides, the telomeres get shorter. When the telomeres become too short, a cell reaches a point when it can't divide anymore and it becomes inactive or dies. This process is associated with aging. But guess what? Exercise has been found to reduce the rate at which telomeres shorten and to increase the rate at which telomeres are repaired, which helps them maintain their length. In either case, exercise appears to be a good way to keep your telomeres in good shape!

- **Enhancement of brainpower.** Even though your brain is not a muscle, physical exercise does strengthen your brain. In fact, research in mice shows that regular exercise increases the number of the energy-producing organelles (mitochondria) not only in muscle cells but in the brain cells as well. This finding suggests that the increase in brain mitochondria may have a role in making the brain more resistant to fatigue as well as being important in fighting mental disorders. Physical exercise also stimulates a process called neurogenesis, a fancy word for the formation of new brain cells (neurons). Exercise can enhance the connections between brain cells, which helps maintain memory and the ability to learn, and reduces the risk of Alzheimer's disease and other dementias, as well as cognitive problems.

AEROBIC EXERCISE VERSUS STRENGTH TRAINING

All exercise is not created equal . . . nor does it benefit the body in the same way. And—no surprise—you need to integrate both aerobic and strength activities into your lifestyle to reap the most life-extending advantages.

Aerobic Exercise

Aerobic exercise, also known as cardiovascular exercise, is physical activity that gets your blood and heart pumping, increases your breathing rate, involves your large muscle groups (e.g., those in your legs), and involves sustained movement. Examples include brisk walking, hiking, stair stepping, aerobic dance, running, swimming, cycling (on the road and stationery), cross-country skiing, rowing, roller skating, in-line or ice skating, water aerobics, and jumping rope.

Choose which aerobic exercises you want to incorporate into your lifestyle. Your age-defying guidelines are as follows:

- Check with your doctor before beginning any new exercise program.

- Choose exercises that you enjoy; that way you will be more likely to continue doing them. If possible, mix it up: brisk walking two days, cycling two days, and aerobics class one day.

- If you have not exercised in a while (and you have your doctor's okay), start slow and gradually increase your time and intensity over a period of several weeks, based on your fitness level.

- Each aerobic exercise session should be at least twenty continuous minutes.

- Strive to do aerobic exercise five to six days a week.

- Do not skip more than two days in a row (unless you are ill or injured).

- Stay hydrated with filtered water.

- Work toward maintaining an intensity level where you are working a bit too hard to carry on a conversation. If you are new to exercise or haven't exercised in a while, work up to this intensity gradually. For example, you could work hard for one minute, then slow down for two, then work hard for another minute and keep alternating.

- Post your exercise plan in a conspicuous place: the front of the refrigerator, on the bathroom mirror, on your dashboard. Write it into your calendar until it becomes a natural part of your day.

You don't need to join a fitness club or gym to participate in aerobic exercise. If you live in an area that is not safe or feasible for exercise, you might exercise at home with videos (you can borrow them from a library, get inexpensive ones at garage sales), along with fitness shows on TV, or use a Wii Fit program. If you live in an apartment or condominium complex that has an exercise room, take advantage of it! Some community centers, churches, and hospitals have free or low-cost exercise or fitness programs for seniors. If there is a mall nearby, see if there is a walking club that meets for regular exercise.

STRENGTH-BUILDING EXERCISES

Even if you have never lifted weights (1) it's never too late to start and (2) yes, you have. Let's address the second phrase first. If you have ever lifted groceries out of the car, carried your grandchild, hoisted a bag of fertilizer out of the shed or garage and carried it into the backyard, or put out the trash, you have lifted weights. So don't be put off by the phrase "lifting weights" and think you can't do it, because chances are, you already have.

You are also never too old to start strength training. In fact, one study reported that among people who averaged 92 years of age strength increased by about 175 percent after they did strength training for only a few minutes per day, three times a week, for one month. They even improved their walking speed and balance enough to retire their walkers and canes. So if your excuse is, "I'm too old to do strength training," forget it.

Strength training is a critical part of an age-defying exercise program for several reasons:

- You lose muscle tone and strength as you age, and performing regular strengthening exercises can curtail that loss so you can function at your very best for as long as possible. You have two basic types of muscles: slow-twitch and fast-twitch. Slow-twitch muscles are used for functions such as walking and bicycling, and they are designed to keep working for long periods of time without getting tired. You call upon your fast-twitch muscles, however, whenever you need to do something that requires a lot of strength, such as opening a stubborn jar of jam or lifting groceries out of your trunk. Unfortunately, fast-twitch muscles are randomly eliminated as people age. This process, called sarcopenia, affects about 45 percent of people. Although strength training cannot totally prevent sarcopenia, it can make a significant difference in your ability to maintain muscle strength.

- Developing lean muscle helps reduce the symptoms and signs of many chronic conditions associated with the aging process, such as arthritis, back pain, depression, diabetes, high blood pressure, and obesity.

- Strength training can help you avoid the possibility
  of falls and resulting fractures, a significant problem among older adults.

Strength Training 101

The American College of Sports Medicine developed
strength-training guidelines specifically for people older
than 50. Their advice is simple: practice strength-building
exercises two to three times a week that address all of the
major muscle groups. The goal is for you to lift an amount
of weight that is heavy enough for you to complete ten to
fifteen repetitions per session before your muscles become
fatigued. For some people, the amount of weight may be
only a few pounds; for others, it may mean using 25- or
30-pound weights—or more. The amount of weight is not
the point: it's what you do with that weight that's important.

Forget the adage "no pain, no gain." Although it is normal to experience sore muscles the day after you do strength
training, you should never feel joint, muscle, or nerve pain.
These are signs that you have gone too far and may have in-
curred tissue damage or strains that can take weeks or even
months to heal. During such downtime you will lose muscle
tone and strength, so preventing injury is a priority.

If you have never done any strength training—and many
people have not—it is critical you speak with your doctor
before you begin. He or she can at least let you know what
you can and should not do and perhaps can refer you to a
physical therapist, personal trainer, or other fitness professional who can develop a program for you. If possible, find
someone who is used to working with someone of your age
and specific needs. Do *not* just walk into a gym and start
using weights and equipment without first getting some professional advice.

Strength-Building Exercises

The following strength exercises are offered as examples only. Please consult your health-care provider or physical therapist to determine the best exercises for your age and state of health.

You will need dumbbells to do these exercises. If you will be using very light weights (1 to 5 lbs.), you can make your own if you don't want to buy them. (See "Making Your Own Dumbbells and Weights" below.)

MAKING YOUR OWN DUMBBELLS AND WEIGHTS

You probably have a few things around your house that can be used as light dumbbells or hand weights. If you plan to work out at home, then no one else needs to know that you use items from your pantry to make hand weights. For example:

- If you are starting out with very light weight, a can of soup or vegetables weighs less than 1 pound and can be held easily in your hands as you do your strength and some stretching exercises.

- If you are ready to move on to something heavier, you can use empty plastic milk, juice, or laundry detergent bottles, because they often have a handle. You can put water into the bottles, weigh them, and then add or subtract water until you reach the desired weight.

- Put sand into old cotton pillowcases to make softer weights.

- Use 1- or 2-pound bags of rice or beans as weights.

- Make beanbags out of material and filled with sand or beans. These make good hand weights.

Shoulder Shrugs (Stabilize Your Shoulders)

- Stand up straight and place your feet slightly apart. Hold hand weights or dumbbells in your hands and place your arms at your sides.

- Inhale and shrug your shoulders up toward your ears as high as you can. Hold this position for several seconds, than exhale and roll your shoulders back while squeezing your shoulder blades together. Hold the squeeze for several seconds, then drop your shoulders back to your starting position. Do 10 times.

Squats (Strengthen Upper Legs)

- Hold the dumbbells in your hands with your palms facing inward.

- Stand with your feet slightly wider than shoulder-width apart and your toes pointed slightly out. Keep your back straight, your knees slightly bent, and your head up.

- Inhale, contract your abdominal muscles, and bend your knees, slowly lowering your body (pretend you are going to sit on a chair). Go down as far as is comfortable, with the goal of reaching a point where your thighs are nearly parallel with the floor.

- Hold the lowest position you can reach for a few seconds, then exhale as you push up with your heels and slowly rise up to your starting position.

- Repeat 8 to 10 times.

Curl Those Biceps (Strengthens the Upper Arms)

- Hold the dumbbells in your hands with your palms up and your arms at your sides.

- Stand with your feet slightly apart and your knees slightly bent.

- Inhale as you contract your abdominal muscles and curl the dumbbells up to your shoulders as you twist your palms so they are facing you when your hands reach your shoulders. Hold this position for a second and exhale as you gradually lower the dumbbells to your starting position.

- Repeat 8 to 10 times.

Rowing with One Arm (Strengthens the Back and Shoulders)

- You will need a workout bench or a sturdy kitchen or dining room armless chair with a flat seat (padded is okay). Kneel on the bench or chair seat with your left knee and place your left hand on the bench or seat as well, supporting your weight.

- Hold a dumbbell in your right hand so your hand is down, palm facing toward your side.

- Inhale and contract your abdominal muscles. Bend your right elbow and gradually raise the dumbbell up to your chest. Keep your elbow high and lift it above your shoulder height. Hold this position for a second, then exhale as you return to the starting position.

- Repeat 8 to 10 times on this side, then repeat with your right knee and hand on the bench or chair seat.

Upper Arm Extensions (Strengthen Back of Upper Arms)

- Hold one dumbbell in both hands, fingers intertwined.

- Stand with your feet slightly apart and your knees slightly bent.

- Inhale as you raise the dumbbell over your head and fully extend your arms.

- Contract your abdominal muscles as you gradually bend your elbows and lower the dumbbell behind your head and neck.

- Try to lower the dumbbell until your forearms are parallel to the floor. Hold this position for a second, then exhale as you gradually raise the dumbbell to your starting position.

- Repeat 8 to 10 times.

Lunges (Strengthen the Legs)

- Hold the dumbbells in each hand with your arms at your sides and your palms facing inward.

- Stand with your feet shoulder-width apart and your back straight, head up, and knees slightly bent.

- Inhale and contract your abdominal muscles as you

step forward with your right foot. Bend both knees so your right thigh is parallel to the floor. Your front knee should be directly above your ankle.

- Hold this position for a second and then exhale as you return to your starting position by pushing off from your front foot.

- Do 8 to 10 repetitions on your right. Then switch sides and do 8 to 10 repetitions on your left foot.

STRETCHING

Stretching doesn't build muscle or improve endurance, but it has other benefits that can help you fight aging. When you stretch, you

- Enhance blood circulation

- Clear your mind

- Reduce the risk of injuries to soft tissue, such as muscle strains and ligament injuries

- Release muscle tension and soreness

- Boost energy

- Improve flexibility

- Increase body awareness, which leads to a better connection between your mind and body and helps make your movements more efficient

- Increase range of motion

- Improve your posture

The National Institute on Aging recommends you stretch after you do your strength and aerobic exercises, but feel free to do stretching exercises more often! On the days you don't do strength-training or cardiovascular exercise, you should at least stretch for about twenty minutes. When you do strength-training and aerobic exercises, your stretching sessions can follow them, or you may want to do your stretching while resting between your different strength-training lifts.

Your role model for stretching is a cat. There's an animal that knows how to stretch: slow, easy, and often. Remember, it's a stretch, not a bounce or a jerking motion. Although you may expect to feel some mild pulling or discomfort when stretching, especially in the beginning, you should not stretch until you feel pain. In fact, there's a two-hour rule of stretching: if you feel worse two hours after stretching, then you stretched too much, so take it easier next time.

Some simple stretching guidelines are:

- **Relax.** This is rule number one when stretching, because if you begin your stretching session feeling uptight, you can easily hurt yourself. Take a few slow, deep breaths before starting your stretching routine. Play some relaxing music while you do your stretches.

- **Warm up.** You need to raise the temperature of your muscles before you stretch them. A good prelude to a stretching session is a warm bath or a short, light walk with your arms swinging freely.

- **Pay attention to what your body is saying to you.** If you feel pain, stop. If a stretch begins to get uncomfortable, back off.

- **Move slowly.** As you move from one stretching position to another, do it slowly, especially if you are changing from a vertical to a horizontal position, or vice versa.

- **Keep breathing.** Healthful breathing is done through the nose, is deep, and causes your belly—not your rib cage—to expand. An effective way to stretch when you have a tight muscle is to inhale first and then exhale as you are stretching.

- **Maintain balance.** In other words, if you do an exercise that stretches your thigh muscles, be sure to do an exercise that tightens them as well. You want to keep everything in balance.

- **Do slow, sustained stretches.** The most effective and safest stretches are those you do slowly and then hold. Avoid bouncing, which can strain or cause tiny tears in your muscle fibers. After your muscles are warmed up, do each stretch two to four times and gradually hold each stretch for a longer period of time. You might begin by holding each stretch for only three to five seconds and, over weeks, extend the time to thirty seconds or more.

- **Expect change.** A stretch you were able to do easily one day may be more difficult on another day. Factors such as how much activity you engaged in the day before, sleeping position, flare-ups of arthritis, and others can influence your ability to stretch. Respect your body and expect changes to occur.

Sample Stretching Exercises

Here are a few stretching exercises for you to consider. Be sure to discuss a stretching program with a knowledgeable individual who can help you choose the stretches best for you. Typically, each stretching exercise should be done three to five times at each session. You will need to hold a towel as part of the stretch in some exercises.

Triceps Stretches (the Muscles in the Back of Your Upper Arms)

- Hold one end of a towel (kitchen towel size) in your right hand.

- Raise your right arm and bend the arm so the towel drapes down your back.

- Take your left hand and arm and reach behind your lower back to grasp the bottom edge of the towel.

- Move your left hand progressively up the towel, which in turn pulls your right arm down. Keep moving your left hand up the towel until your hands touch or you cannot go any farther comfortably. Hold the stretch for five to thirty seconds.

- Repeat using the left hand and arm to drape the towel over your back.

- Repeat the exercise 3 to 5 times each session.

Hamstring Stretches (the Muscles in the Back of Your Thighs)

- Stand behind a sturdy chair and hold on to the back of the chair with both hands. Keep your legs straight.

- Bend forward from your hips (not your waist) while keeping your back and shoulders straight until your upper body is parallel to the floor.

- Hold this position for five to thirty seconds. You should feel a stretch in the back of your thighs.

- Slowly rise to the starting position. Repeat 3 to 5 times.

Quadriceps Stretches (the Muscles in the Front of Your Thighs)

- Lie on the floor on your left side. Your hips should be aligned so the right one is directly above the left one.

- Place your head on a pillow or your left hand.

- Bend your right knee and reach with your right hand until you grab onto your right heel. If this is too much of a stretch, loop a belt over your right foot and hold on to the belt.

- Pull gently with your hand (or the belt) until the front of your right thigh feels stretched. Hold the stretch for five to thirty seconds.

- Now turn over and lie on your right side and repeat the exercise with the other leg. Repeat the exercise 3 to 5 times on each side.

Hip Rotations (Stretch the Outer Muscles of Your Thighs and Hips)

- **Warning:** If you have had a hip replacement, do not do this stretching exercise.

- Lie on your back on the floor and bend your knees so your feet are flat on the floor.

- Relax your shoulders on the floor and keep them on the floor throughout the exercise.

- With your knees bent and together, gently lower your legs to one side as far as you can without causing discomfort. Hold the stretch for five to thirty seconds.

- Slowly return your legs to the upright starting position.

- Repeat the stretch to the other side.

- Repeat the stretch on each side 3 to 5 times.

BALANCE AND HAND-EYE COORDINATION

Preservation of your balance and hand-eye coordination is critical as you age to help you maintain optimal functioning. Many fun leisure activities are especially helpful for promoting and maintaining balance and/or hand-eye coordination, so if you haven't enjoyed any of these opportunities, now may be the time to explore some of them. These are activities you can include each week as part of your leisure time physical exercise. Some examples include badminton, bowling, croquet, dancing, Frisbee, golf, horseshoes, karate, Pilates, racquetball, tai chi (studies show tai chi can significantly improve balance), tennis, volleyball, and yoga.

An activity as simple as playing catch with your children or grandchildren helps hand-eye coordination. Want a real challenge (and also to impress your friends and family)? Learn to juggle. Begin with two tennis balls and work your way up to four. Juggling takes lots of practice, but it is an excellent way to develop hand-eye coordination.

If you have access to a Wii game system, there are activities you can play to promote balance and coordination. Many of the video games on the market are also an excellent way to play while improving your hand-eye coordination.

You can also easily incorporate balance and hand-eye coordination exercises into your daily routine. Balance exercises can be done while standing in line at the store, watching TV, doing the dishes, during a break at work, or just about anywhere. Here are a few examples:

Shifting Weight

- Stand with your feet hip-width apart and your weight evenly distributed on both legs.

- Shift your weight to your right side, then lift your left foot off the ground.

- Hold this position as long as you can without flailing your arms. If you can only stay balanced for a few seconds, that's fine; you will get better with practice. Your goal is to hold the position for 30 seconds.

- Return to your starting position and repeat with the other leg.

- Repeat the exercise 3 to 5 times on each side.

Single Leg Bends

- Stand with your feet hip-width apart and your weight evenly distributed on both legs.

- Place your hands on your hips.

- Lift your left leg off the ground and bend it back at the knee.

- Hold this position for at least 5 seconds, with a goal of 30.

- Return to the starting position and repeat with the other leg.

- Repeat the exercise 3 to 5 times on each side.

Side and Dumbbell Raises

- Stand with your feet hip-width apart and your weight evenly distributed on both legs. Hold a dumbbell in your right hand and raise your arm until it is perpendicular to the ground.

- Lift your right leg off the ground and bend it back at the knee.

- Hold this position for at least 5 seconds, with a goal of 30.

- Return to the starting position and repeat on the other side.

WHAT THE STUDIES SAY

One thing is for sure: there is no shortage of studies or opinions about the benefits of exercise for extending life. One thing all the studies have in common: none of them say being sedentary adds years to your life. You may be surprised, however, at how little effort you need to exert to lengthen your life span by just a few years. Add more exercise, say experts, and you add even more years.

For example: A 2011 study in Taiwan evaluated the amount of exercise performed by more than four hundred thousand adults between 1996 and 2008. Then they calculated the risk of death among the active adults and compared it to the inactive adults. They found that adults who exercised fifteen minutes a day had a life expectancy that was three years longer than that of adults who were sedentary and a 14 percent reduced risk of dying. For every additional fifteen minutes of exercise per day beyond the original fifteen minutes, the adults gained another 4 percent reduced risk of dying. These results are important because they not only support the benefits of exercise for extending life but also apply to both men and women *and* people with risks for cardiovascular disease, such as obesity, high blood pressure, and high cholesterol.

On the other end of the couch, researchers in Australia found that watching TV or videos for an average of six hours a day could shorten your life by nearly five years when compared with people who don't watch TV at all. They even broke it down by minutes: for every hour you watch TV after age 25, you lose twenty-two minutes off your life span. These findings suggest that watching TV is comparable to other risk factors, such as lack of exercise and obesity.

However, I have a solution for those of you who watch TV or DVDs at least an hour or so: if you do your strength-training exercises and/or use a treadmill or other exercise machine while watching TV, you cancel out the coach potato effect!

The bottom line is, if you make various types of exercise a part of your life, you have a very good chance of adding healthy, quality years to your life.

STEP 4

Take Control of Your Health Care

"It's my body and my health, and I think I have the right to make my own health-care decisions." More and more people are expressing this sentiment and, more important, they are doing something about it. This chapter can help you take the actions to gain control over your health-care decisions.

The state of health care in the United States (and in other countries) is frustrating, complex, and, in many ways, inadequate, despite the presence of much high-tech equipment and many procedures. Health care is out of reach for many Americans, given the costs (even with insurance) of medications and procedures, the number of doctors not accepting new patients, and a decline in general practitioners and specialists in certain areas. These and other factors make it all the more necessary for you to take control of your own health care as much as possible.

One thing that has made taking control of your own health care possible is increased access to important, relevant health information on the Internet. This access comes with caveats, however. For example, not every Web site provides accurate information, so you need to know how to recognize the sites that are safe. (There are tips in this chapter.) Another caution is to gather research from several sources—similar to getting a second and third opinion.

You may also need some help interpreting the information you gather, which means you will need to have a trustworthy, knowledgeable health-care provider to turn to.

Someday, in the not-so-distant future, everyone should be able to track their health and aging status with a technique called telomere testing. Scientists are working on this process, which will allow you to get information on your overall health on a cellular level and a glimpse into your future health based on the status of those champions of natural cellular aging—your telomeres.

For now, however, you have to rely on other sources at your disposal, and that's the topic of discussion in this chapter: information you can use to take control of your own preventive health care.

AN OUNCE OR TWO OF PREVENTION

The best medicine is the need for no medicine at all, and one way to avoid medication and medical procedures, or detect problems early, is to take preventive steps. Those steps include the following:

- Get recommended screenings to check your general health and the status of specific parts of your body (e.g., breasts, bones, prostate, et cetera).

- Know which immunizations are recommended for adults.

- Identify who and where to turn to when you need professional help.

- Keep accurate personal health records, including diaries when necessary (e.g., if you are monitoring your blood sugar or weight-loss program). This is especially critical when you need to consult medical professionals.

- Follow healthful advice concerning diet, exercise, stress, drug use (alcohol, tobacco, medications), and sleep.

This chapter involves a discussion of these points; the last one is also covered in detail in other steps in this book. The point is, if you monitor your own health, you will be an informed, empowered health-care consumer and an active participant in your own health, well-being, and longevity.

HEALTH SCREENINGS

Health screenings are tests or exams that are performed to find a condition before symptoms become apparent. A major goal of such screenings is to detect and identify diseases or conditions early enough so they are easier to treat and treatment will be more effective. Although early screening tests have not been developed for every disease, many such tests are available for common conditions, all of which are frequently seen in people as they age. They include screenings for breast cancer, cervical cancer, colon cancer, prostate cancer, diabetes, and osteoporosis. In addition, there are other screening tests that are usually reserved for individuals who have certain risk factors for Alzheimer's disease, heart disease, lung diseases, and liver diseases, among others.

Here is an overview of the common screening tests recommended for adults at various stages of their lives. If you have health insurance, check to see if it covers screening tests. If you do not have health insurance, you will need to pay for the tests on your own or look for low-cost or free screenings that are periodically offered by different health organizations and held in community centers, medical facilities, and senior centers around the country.

Hint: Often there are free screenings offered in the month named for a specific disease or condition. For example, October is National Breast Cancer Awareness Month and every year there are scores of opportunities in towns and cities across the United States for uninsured and underinsured women to get a free or low-cost mammogram. The story is similar for cervical cancer, prostate cancer, and diabetes. The secret is, *be proactive*. Look for these opportunities in your area: check hospitals, clinics, the public health department, centers for the aging, health fairs, senior centers, and the Internet for offerings from the American Cancer Association, the American Diabetes Association, and the Centers for Disease Control and Prevention.

Breast Cancer

Experts still disagree on the optimal schedule for mammograms. Depending on whether you listen to the American Cancer Society, the National Cancer Institute, or the U.S. Preventive Services Task Force, among others, you will get different recommendations for when to get a mammogram. Each woman should consider all the options and her family's cancer and medical history, as well as her own health and her doctor's advice, before making a decision. Generally:

- Women should begin doing a breast self-exam every month starting in their twenties.

- A clinical breast exam (by a medical professional) should be done every three years for women in their twenties and thirties and yearly for women 40 and older.

- Mammograms are recommended starting at age 40 or 50 and continuing at varying intervals, depending on the source, but generally every one to two years until age 74, when you may choose to cease this screening.

- The American Cancer Society recommends that some women who have a family history, a genetic tendency, or other risk factors be screened with magnetic resonance imaging (MRI) in addition to mammograms. Only about 2 percent of women fall into this high-risk category.

Cervical Cancer

Screening for cervical cancer involves having a Pap test, which currently must be done by a health-care provider. However, home-based tests are under development and may be available in the near future. The recommended screening schedule is as follows:

- First screening should be about three years after first vaginal intercourse, but no later than age 21 years. Screening should be yearly if the regular Pap test is used or every two years if the newer liquid-based test is used.

- Beginning at age 30, if you have had three normal Pap test results in a row, screening can change to every 2 to 3 years with either Pap test.

- Women age 70 and older who have had 3 or more normal Pap test results in a row and no abnormal results within the last 10 years may choose to stop screening.

- Women who have had a total hysterectomy can stop screenings for cervical cancer unless their surgery was done as a treatment for cervical cancer or precancer.

Colon Cancer

Screening for colon cancer is recommended beginning at age 50 for both women and men. The two basic types of screening tests available are invasive and noninvasive. The invasive tests are designed to detect polyps and cancer and include:

- Flexible sigmoidoscopy, which is recommended every five years

- Double-contrast barium enema, every five years

- Virtual colonoscopy, every five years

- Colonoscopy, every ten years

If the results of any of the first three tests are positive, a colonoscopy should be done. Your other choice is a noninvasive test, which is designed primarily to find cancer, not polyps. You can purchase these tests at a drugstore or online and take the test at home by following the instructions on the package. If the results are positive, you should have a colonoscopy. The tests include:

- Yearly fecal occult blood test (gFOBT)

- Yearly fecal immunochemical test (FIT)

- Stool DNA test (sDNA), no set interval

The tests designed to detect both polyps and early-stage cancer are typically preferred by physicians. If you do not have insurance, if you are not willing to have an invasive test, or if you want to handle testing on your own, that is your choice, but you should discuss the risks and benefits with your physician.

Prostate Cancer

Debate surrounds the benefits and risks of prostate cancer screening using the PSA (prostate-specific antigen) test, because there is much conflicting information regarding whether the potential benefits of testing outweigh the harm of testing and subsequent treatment. Generally, starting at age 50 (or 45 if there is a history of prostate cancer in the family or you are African American), you should discuss the pros and cons of testing with your physician. If you decide to be screened, your doctor will also do a digital rectal exam as part of the screening process. How often you choose to be tested will depend on your PSA score.

Prostate cancer screenings are frequently offered free of charge or for a minimal fee during Prostate Cancer Awareness Week or other times during the year. The Prostate Conditions Education Council, for example, offers hundreds of free screening opportunities throughout the year (http://www .prostateconditions.org/).

Diabetes

The American Diabetes Association recommends adults begin routine screening around age 45, which involves a fasting blood sugar test (a simple blood test taken after fasting). Testing is available through your health-care provider, but it is also often offered free or for minimal charge at health fairs, clinics, and other venues. Blood testing at such events typically does not require people to fast beforehand, but you should fast, if possible, for ten to twelve hours before the test. Subsequent screening will be recommended if your test result is 126 mg/dL or higher, which indicates a diagnosis of diabetes. An ideal reading is between 80 and 120 mg/dL, although you should have your blood sugar level checked once a year or so if your reading is between 100 and 125 mg/dL. You should also have your blood sugar taken at least once a year if you are overweight, have a family history of diabetes, or have other medical problems often associated with diabetes, such as heart disease, high blood pressure, or high cholesterol.

Osteoporosis

Osteoporosis is a common disease that mostly affects women in their menopausal and postmenopausal years. It is a silent disease, which means it presents no symptoms, and so the only ways people know they have osteoporosis is if they (1) fall and/or otherwise break a bone and the osteoporosis is discovered on X-rays or (2) they have a bone mineral density test.

A bone mineral density test or screening should be done if you fit into any of the following categories: woman age 65 or older or man 70 or older; or woman younger than 65 or man age 50 to 70 who has risk factors for osteoporosis, such as chronic rheumatoid arthritis or kidney disease, early menopause, history of hormone treatment, smoking, strong family history of osteoporosis, having suffered a bone fracture caused by normal activity, or having used corticosteroids daily for more than three months.

It is possible to get a simple bone density scan using a portable machine as part of a health fair or community screening event, which may be low cost or free, and in some doctors' offices. Portable scanners check the density of your heel or wrist, but a more reliable reading is done by a central DEXA (dual-energy X-ray absorptiometry) scan, which scans your lower spine and hip and typically is done in a hospital or large clinic. You and your health-care provider can discuss your need for future scans, depending on the results of your scan.

Blood Pressure

Blood pressure is an important factor to monitor because high blood pressure has no symptoms and left untreated can lead to a stroke, a heart attack, kidney failure, or heart failure. It is also a factor you can check at home using a reliable blood pressure monitoring device (available through pharmacies/drugstores and medical supply houses), or you can have readings done at your health-care provider's office, a clinic, a health fair, or similar venues. If you check your own blood pressure, do it at the same time of the day each time and take two readings several minutes apart. Blood pressure values are as follows:

- Normal blood pressure is defined as less than 120 (systolic) over less than 80 (diastolic). If your BP is normal, check it once every two years.

- Prehypertension is 120-139 over 80-89, and you should have it checked at least once a year.

- Stage 1 (140-159 over 90-99) and stage 2 hypertension (160+ over 100+) should be monitored closely by your physician.

Cholesterol

Cholesterol screening is done to help identify the risk of developing heart disease. High total cholesterol is a risk factor for cardiovascular disease, as are high levels of low-density lipoprotein (LDL) and triglycerides and low levels of high-density lipoprotein (HDL) cholesterol. You should have your blood cholesterol levels checked beginning at age 40 and at least once every five years (or earlier and more often if you have diabetes, high blood pressure, or a family history of heart disease or if you smoke). If you are already being treated for high cholesterol, you should be checked several times a year. The screening is simple: a complete lipid panel—total, HDL, and LDL cholesterol plus triglycerides—can be determined from a small blood sample.

You may have been to a health fair where they checked cholesterol levels, and this type of testing is okay for total cholesterol. However, it is best to have all your lipid levels checked. Home test kits for cholesterol are also available, and they, too, can be okay for self-monitoring. However, if any of your factors are abnormal, it is best to have them checked by a health professional.

- Normal cholesterol: less than 200 mg/dL

- Borderline high: 200–239 mg/dL

- High cholesterol: 240 mg/dL and higher

- LDL: 100–129 mg/dL is ideal, while <120 mg/dL is best for people at risk for heart disease

- HDL: >60 mg/dL is ideal, while <50 mg/dL for women and <40 mg/dL for men is poor

- Triglycerides: <150 mg/dL is desirable

Thyroid Disease

Screening for thyroid disease is controversial, but I mention it because thyroid conditions are often overlooked in women as they grow older and detecting any problem can have a significant effect on health and longevity. The American Thyroid Association recommends that everyone older than 35 years be screened with a TSH (thyroid stimulating hormone) test every five years, while the American Association of Clinical Endocrinologists recommends that all women be tested for hypothyroidism (underactive thyroid) by age 50 and sooner if they have a family history of thyroid disease. There's no home test for this one, so you'll need to see a health-care provider.

Eye Exams

Screening for age-related eye diseases—cataracts, glaucoma, macular degeneration, and presbyopia (a progressive inability to focus on near objects)—should begin at age 40. Your eyes are the windows to your soul—and to other health issues as well—so early screening may also uncover early signs of diabetes, high blood pressure, and other conditions. Once you've been screened for age-related eye conditions, you should get an eye exam every two years if you don't wear corrective lenses, in which case yearly is recommended. Yearly eye exams should begin for all adults at ages 60 to 65 to monitor any vision changes and eye diseases.

VACCINATIONS

Vaccinations are not just for children, so as an adult you'll be asked to roll up your sleeve a few times should you decide to get the recommended shots. In addition to the following vaccinations, you may need other vaccines if you are traveling out of the country. The Centers for Disease Control and Prevention offers information on required and recommended vaccines when traveling abroad. (See http://wwwnc.cdc.gov/travel/page/vaccinations.htm.)

Here at home, however, the following vaccines are recommended:

- **Flu vaccine.** This vaccine is now recommended yearly for anyone 6 months of age and older. If you are healthy, not pregnant, and younger than 50, you can choose between the intranasally administered live, attenuated vaccine (FluMist) and the inactivated vaccine. If you are older than 65, you can get the standard flu vaccine or the high-dose (Fluzone) vaccine.

- **Pneumonia (pneumococcal polysaccharide).** You should consider this vaccine if you smoke or if you have chronic lung disease (including asthma), diabetes, chronic liver disease, chronic alcoholism, chronic cardiovascular disease, any immunocompromising condition (e.g., chronic renal failure, nephritic syndrome), or cochlear implants. Anyone who lives in a nursing home or long-term care facility also should get a pneumococcal vaccination. In November 2011, the Vaccines and Related Biological Products Advisory Committee of the Food and Drug Administration voted to expand the indication for the pneumococcal vaccine Prevnar 13 to adults aged 50 years and older. This recommendation was given because pneumococcal infections "remain an important cause of morbidity and mortality among older adults," stated the FDA's document.

- **Tetanus, diphtheria, pertussis.** All adults aged 19 to 64 who have not already received the tetanus/diphtheria/pertussis vaccination and have not received a Td booster immunization in the last ten years should get a single dose of Tdap. Adults older than 65 who have not had a Td booster in the last ten years should receive Td.

- **Herpes zoster, otherwise known as shingles.** A vaccine against this often-debilitating condition hit the market in 2006. The Centers for Disease Control and Prevention recommends the shingles vaccine (ZOSTAVAX) for individuals age 60 years and older as a preventive measure, regardless of whether they had chicken pox or not. The vaccine is not designed to treat active shingles or postherpetic neuralgia (pain that persists after the rash of shingles has disappeared). Before the vaccine was introduced to the market, clinical research indicated that ZOSTAVAX reduced the risk of shingles by 51 percent and the risk of postherpetic neuralgia by 67 percent. The vaccine proved most effective for people age 60 to 69, but it is also helpful for people who are older. The vaccine appears to be effective for at least six years, but it could last longer. The vaccine was designed as a onetime injection. If you have already had shingles and never received the vaccine, you can get it to help prevent recurrence of the disease.

BE PREPARED

Sometimes surprises are great: surprise parties, a surprise raise, a surprise rebate. A health emergency, however, is the type of surprise that isn't welcome. You can help take some of the anxiety out of a medical emergency by being prepared. Here are some things you can do:

- **Carry emergency information with you.** Everyone should have a card in his or her wallet or purse that contains necessary information in case of a medical emergency. It's also important that you update the information whenever there is a change. Your wallet-sized card should contain: your name and date of birth, who to contact in case of emergency (name and phone), doctor name and phone, list of medications and doses (including over-the-counter, prescription, and supplements), any allergies you have to medications or other substances, blood type, medical condition(s) (e.g., diabetes, epilepsy, high blood pressure, heart disease), and medical and dental insurance numbers.

- **Keep emergency information at home.** The same information you carry in your wallet or purse should be posted on your refrigerator or at another prominent place in your home so emergency personnel can easily see it. Why? Assume you will be unable to provide the critical information the professionals will need to know once they reach you. Emergency medical workers know to look for such information in a home.

- **Take a first-aid/CPR course.** The American Red Cross, local hospitals, colleges, emergency medical facilities, and community centers typically offer first-aid and/or CPR training. The information and skills you learn from these courses can prove invaluable, even lifesaving, for yourself and your family.

- **Keep a personal health record (PHR).** You can create your own PHR, or your health-care provider or insurer or a commercial supplier of PHRs may be your choice. If you are taking much of your health care into your own hands, make sure you add relevant information to your record. For example, your primary-care physician has a medical file on you, but if you regularly check your own blood pressure at home with a home monitor, you should keep a record of those readings. If you take advantage of a free or low-cost mammogram at a local clinic, the staff will ask for your doctor's name so they can send the results to him or her. However, you can also ask that the results be sent to you, and you should keep the results as part of your PHR. (See "Personal Health Records 101" below for more information.)

- **Know your family medical history.** This information, along with your personal health record, can be invaluable if medical professionals ever need in-depth information that may have an impact on diagnosis and treatment decisions. Make a point to collect information about your parents, grandparents, and siblings.

Personal Health Records 101

There are a wide range of products available to help you create your own PHR and actively monitor your health. You may choose to store your information on a thumb drive or disc, or you can take advantage of one of the Internet-based services you can access from your home computer that will allow you to store and retrieve your health information at will. Some PHR tools are free, while you must purchase others or pay a subscription fee to use them. Explore your options and then decide which method works best for you.

To get started, here are some tips:

- Request a copy of your health records from all of your health-care providers: primary-care physician, specialists, eye doctor, dentist, chiropractor, and alternative-medicine practitioners. Contact each provider and ask how you can most easily get this information from him or her. These providers may also have their own plan for helping their patients create a PHR, and you may choose to receive assistance from them. If your medical records are maintained by your health plan, you will need to contact the organization's customer service department.

- You may need to get a form called an "authorization for the release of information" from your health-care providers. Ask if this form is required.

- Once you have accumulated the necessary information, choose the type of PHR that best suits your needs. You may simply put everything in a three-ring binder with separate tabs for each type of medical care, or you may want to use an electronic version of a PHR. You can also include family medical history information in your PHR so everything will be in one convenient place.

- Bring your PHR with you whenever you visit a health-care provider so you will keep updating your information and the providers will have access to anything they may not have in their records.

DON'T KEEP YOUR MEDICAL WISHES A SECRET

Along with keeping a PHR, you should also do two other tasks: complete advance directives (a living will) and assign a trusted individual with your medical or health-care power of attorney. A living will is a document that describes your wishes regarding treatment if you are unable to speak for yourself; for example, if you have a serious accident or suffer a stroke. Because accidents can happen to anyone at any age, living wills are not just for older adults, and having one available can eliminate confusion and disagreement about your preferred treatment.

Your health-care power of attorney should be given to an individual you choose to make medical decisions for you if you are not able to do so. (Note that this is not the same as a financial power of attorney.) Assigning a health-care power of attorney is a critical part of controlling your own health-care planning and maintaining control over your health-care wishes as laid out in your living will.

The individual you choose does not have to be a family member: he or she should be someone mature, clear thinking, and who you trust will carry out your wishes and desires. Thus it is important to choose someone whose philosophy about health-care and medical procedures matches yours as closely as possible. This individual should also know where to find your PHR in case of an emergency and you cannot communicate the information to your health-care providers. Although it is more convenient if the person lives nearby, it's more important that the person be someone you trust.

Here are a few things you should know about advance directives/a living will:

- You don't need a lawyer to create an advance directive. You can get the necessary forms free, online, and complete them yourself. The document becomes legally valid *only* after it has been signed in front of the necessary witnesses.

- The laws governing advance directives are not the same in each state, so you should have advance directives that comply with your state's law.

- If you live in one state for six months of the year and in another for six months, you should have an advance directive for each state. If you are traveling and have an accident in a state for which you do not have an advance directive and your injuries are such that the person who has your health-care power of attorney would normally be consulted, the state in which the accident occurred may or may not honor your advance directives. For your protection, it is best to have an advance directive for any state in which you plan to spend a significant amount of time.

- Advance directives do not expire. If you make a new advance directive, it invalidates the older one.

- Emergency medical technicians are not allowed to honor advance directives or medical powers of attorney. After they have stabilized a patient for transfer to a hospital, a physician must evaluate the patient before advance directives can be honored.

- Review your advance directives occasionally to make sure they still reflect your wishes. If you want to make changes, complete a new document, which you can do for no charge using online forms.

You should also consider if you want a Do Not Resuscitate (DNR) order, which is a request to not have cardiopulmonary resuscitation if your heart stops or if you stop breathing. An advance directive does not include a DNR order; it is a separate request your doctor can order on your medical chart.

FINDING COMPETENT HEALTH CARE

Is there a doctor in the house? Is it a doctor you know and trust? Finding competent health-care providers, be they conventional or alternative practitioners, can be a challenge, especially as the medical landscape keeps changing in the United States. These changes can be particularly trouble-

some for older adults, who may find it more difficult to lo-
cate doctors who accept Medicare or who will take new
patients, and for people of any age when they are trying to
find a practitioner whom they can trust. Oftentimes health-
care seekers are limited by their insurance plans when it
comes to service providers or the types of services that are
included. All of these factors can be frustrating.

Still, there are some basic questions you should ask yourself and factors you should consider when looking for one
or more competent health-care providers or even if you are
reevaluating those you have right now:

- **What do you need?** Do you need a general internist or family practitioner, or would you prefer
  someone who handles arthritis or cardiovascular
  conditions? Some internists have additional training in these and other areas, but you may need a
  specialist along with your primary doctor. Women
  often choose a gynecologist to serve as their primary doctor, but you may reach a point where having a dedicated internist in addition to your
  gynecologist serves you better.

- **What are your choices?** Whether you have a
  health plan with a provider list from which you can
  choose or you don't have insurance and you must
  choose from doctors in your area, identify a list of,
  say, internists with a specialty in rheumatic diseases or general practitioners within a 10-mile ra-
  dius.

- **Check qualifications.** Once you have selected several physicians, check with your state medical board
  to make sure they are licensed and have no disciplinary actions against them. (Just because a doctor
  is part of an insurance plan doesn't mean he or she
  passes these two tests.) If you have a health plan,
  check to see if it provides information on individual

physicians, such as a list of high-performance doctors or those who focus on specific conditions such as diabetes or back pain.

- **Check convenience.** Call the offices of the doctors you have picked and ask questions of the office staff. Most of these individuals are extremely busy, so if they cannot answer your questions when you call ask for the best time to call back. You might begin with: "Before I make an appointment, I have a few questions."
  - What type of health insurance does the doctor accept? What other types of payment does the doctor accept? If you do not have insurance, you may be able to negotiate for a reduced or sliding fee. A community health center or clinic may be a better choice for services if you are uninsured. You can find services in your area by contacting the Health Resources and Services Administration (http://www.hrsa.gov/index.html).
  - Does the office file the insurance claims for me?
  - With which hospital is the doctor associated?
  - Is the doctor board certified? (You can check a doctor's certification with the American Board of Medical Specialties (www.abms.org) and at Web sites such as www.healthgrades.com.
  - Is the doctor part of a group practice? Who are the other doctors and what are their specialties?
  - If my doctor was not available, who would see me?
  - Are lab work and X-rays performed in the office or will I need to go to another location?
  - How long is the typical office visit?
  - How long is the typical wait time?
  - Where is the office located and is there parking?

- Does the doctor have weekend and evening hours?
- Is it possible to get a same-day appointment for urgent care?

- **Check out the doctor's Web site**. Many doctors and especially group practices maintain a Web site where you can get much of the information you need. Some doctors even post video clips of themselves and their staff, so you can get an idea of their personalities. (It used to be much easier to arrange a "get-to-know-you" meeting with a physician, but in today's world that is rarely possible. Because doctors are so busy and spend a minimum amount of time with patients, your introductory meeting will likely be blended into your first appointment, so be prepared.)

- **Prepare for your first appointment.** Once you have chosen a doctor and made your first appointment, be sure to bring your personal health records with you. Be prepared to ask questions. (Write them down so you don't forget them.)

- **Evaluate your visit.** Did you feel comfortable with the doctor? Did he or she answer your questions? Did you feel rushed? Were you treated with respect? If you are uncertain about this doctor, you may want to switch to another physician.

PROTECT YOUR HEALTH INFORMATION

Medical identify theft is big business—and not the type of business you want to happen to you. Part of your effort to control your own health care should include protecting your health information from getting into the hands of individuals who can use it to submit false bills to insurance companies, medical suppliers, or other entities or get paid medical care on your dime and your insurance. Has your medical information been compromised? According to the Federal Trade Commission, the answer may be "yes" if you experience any of the following:

- You get a bill for medical services or products you did not receive.

- You see medical collection notices on your credit report that are not yours.

- A debt collector contacts you about medical bills that are not yours.

- Your insurance provider denies a claim you made because they say you've reached your limit on benefits (and you know this is not true).

- You are denied insurance because your medical records show a disease or condition you do not have.

You can reduce the chance your medical information will be jeopardized if you:

- Are cautious of any "free" health products or services.

- Shred your health insurance forms, prescription statements, and doctor statements.

- Review every bill and statement you receive and check your medical records for inaccuracies.

- Never give your health information to anyone you don't know. Your doctor's office may ask you to e-mail information—verify by phone before you send anything.

RELIABLE HEALTH INFORMATION
ON THE INTERNET

Access to the Internet has opened the floodgates when it comes to health-related information. Yet not only is it easy to drown in the deluge of data, but you must also be wary of what you reach for in terms of a life preserver. In short, know the waters in which you swim and always discuss your findings and questions with a knowledgeable health-care practitioner before you take any action.

Generally, you can expect to find reliable health information on Web sites that are run by a federal agency, accredited hospitals and educational institutions, national or international health organizations (e.g., the National Cancer Institute, the American Geriatrics Society, the World Health Organization), textbooks and Web sites (e.g., *The Merck Manual* and *UpToDate Patient Information*), and well-recognized health experts. That does not mean, however, that countless numbers of other smaller, even obscure Web sites don't have valuable information, but you should check their credentials.

So, to help you decide if a Web site is reliable, here are some questions you should have answered. Regardless of what you find, however, the information does not replace medical advice from your health-care provider and you should discuss it with him or her.

- Who sponsors the site?

- Is the site primarily trying to sell you something?

- Who produces and maintains the site? Look for an "About Us" link.

- What credentials does the author (or authors) of the Web site have? Don't take the Web site's word for it: search for the experts listed on the Web site and see what information you find.

- Is the information presented on the Web site backed up with references? A common practice is for a Web site to be peppered with phrases like "studies show" and "researchers say," yet no reference list is offered. If references are listed, spot-check them: sometimes they are inaccurate or false.

- Does the Web site have a way for you to contact the producer or authors?

- Does the information seem to be biased or credible?

- Does the Web site have links to other Web sites? Are the links active and up-to-date?

- Is the information on the Web site dated? When was the site produced, last modified or updated?

- Does the Web site have a privacy policy? Do you understand how the Web site might use any information you provide?

- Can you access information on the Web site without revealing personal information? (A Web site may ask for your e-mail address so you can get a newsletter or updates.)

- Is the information provided on the Web site easy to understand?

- Is the Web site easy to navigate?

- Does the Web site have the HONcode (Health On the Net Foundation) seal of approval? This seal should appear somewhere on the home page of the Web site, usually at the bottom. The Health On the Net Foundation is a nonprofit, nongovernmental organization, accredited to the Economic and Social

Council of the United Nations, that promotes and guides medical- or health-related Web sites and helps ensure the information is reliable and meets ethical standards.

STEP 5

Keep Your Brain Young

Your mind and body are intimately connected: whatever affects one also impacts the other. Therefore, as you strive to keep your body as young and healthy as possible, you also need to nourish your mind. Thus far the steps in this book have focused on maintaining a youthful body: choosing nutritious food, maintaining a healthy weight, participating in physical exercise, and gaining self-control of your health care. You may have noticed, however, that elements of every one of the steps can also apply, directly or indirectly, to keeping your brain young, too.

So now it's time to *focus* on your brain: how to flex your neurons (brain cells) and exercise your mind to prevent memory loss, enhance brainpower, and keep your brain vibrant and functioning to its fullest capacity. And when your mind is functioning at its best there's a positive side effect on your overall health as well.

You might remember the commercial slogan about a mind being a terrible thing to waste, and this is true at any age. It is also true that as you get older you still have a great capacity to learn. Yes, you *can* teach an old dog new tricks! This chapter offers suggestions on how you can keep your brain young as well as how to incorporate these activities into your lifestyle and, I hope, make some of them habits that will reward you with years of physical, emotional, and spiritual well-being.

CAN YOU REALLY ENHANCE YOUR BRAINPOWER?

For many years, doctors and researchers believed that when the human body stopped developing, which is when people reach their early twenties, the human brain also ceased making new neurons (nerve cells that are the basic building blocks of the nervous system) as well as forming any new vital connections between neurons in the brain. Essentially they were saying, once you reached your late twenties your brain had peaked and it was all downhill from there, albeit a slow decline.

Fortunately, they were wrong. The human brain *can* continue making new neurons until the day you die, but as with the muscles in your arms and legs, if you don't nourish and exercise them, they won't thrive and keep on working well for you. Therefore, if you want to stay younger and smarter as you add years to your life, you need to continously interact with your world mentally and physically to preserve and enhance your brainpower. When you mentally stimulate your brain, you protect it against cognitive decline, much like physical exercise protects against loss of muscle strength and tone.

That's not to say that those who have a disease such as Alzheimer's or another form of dementia don't experience severe mental decline. But most age-related loss in memory and other mental activities is the result of a lack of mental stimulation. Researchers from the Albert Einstein College of Medicine in New York, for example, found that older adults who kept mentally active reduced their risk of dementia by as much as 75 percent compared with their peers who did not stimulate their brains. Dare I say it: use it or lose it! Even people who have dementia can benefit from exercising their brain.

WHAT HELPS KEEPS YOUR BRAIN YOUNG?

- Eat nutritious food: Step 1.

- Maintain a healthy weight: Step 2.

- Participate in routine physical exercise: Step 3.

- Get an adequate amount of sleep: Step 5.

- Manage your stress: Step 9.

- Don't smoke: Step 8.

- Limit yourself to a moderate amount of alcohol: Step 8.

- Maintain social interactions on a regular basis: Step 7.

- Avoid environmental toxins: Step 8.

When you continue to challenge yourself and learn new things, you prompt your brain to make new connections that allow your cells to communicate with one another, which in turn helps your brain retrieve and store information, even as you age. Notice the important words here: "challenge" and "new." Exercising your brain to stay smarter longer requires that you do things that broaden your knowledge and force you to think, solve problems, use your memory, and come up with new ideas.

The number of ways you can stimulate your mind are too numerous to count or describe here. However, this chapter can act as a spark to motivate you to try different activities and develop new habits and behaviors that will challenge your brain. The hope is that you will then incorporate those that interest you most into your lifestyle.

LEARN SOMETHING NEW

Several exciting studies have reported that people who know more than one language appear to have some protection against developing Alzheimer's disease. In fact, in one of the latest studies published in *Cortex* researchers reported they had found physical evidence (on computed tomography [CT] scans of patients' brains) that people with probable Alzheimer's who are able to speak more than one language showed twice as much brain damage as people who could speak only one language before they showed symptoms of Alzheimer's disease. This finding indicates that those who are bilingual have built up and strengthened their brain's ability to resist or fight off the damage that can lead to dementia.

These findings have implications for people other than those who develop dementia, because they offer support for other studies that indicate keeping your mind active is an effective way to stay mentally sharp and focused. People who speak more than one language, for example, must be able to mentally switch back and forth between the two and keep them straight in their minds; thus they are challenging their brains. When you challenge your brain, you help form new neural connections and essentially strengthen your mind.

I'm not saying you have to learn a new language, but if you do you may not only help guard your brain against dementia but also open doors of opportunity. Knowing a second language may allow you to read literature in another language, communicate with people you may never have approached before, or make you feel more comfortable when traveling to another country. Some people find that learning to read a new language, rather than becoming proficient at speaking it as well, is both challenging and satisfying, because it allows them to read and even help translate letters and other written items.

Opportunities to learn new hobbies or activities or even start a new career are all around you: on the Internet, at community centers, libraries, schools, businesses, and churches, on DVDs and TV. When you pursue new challenges, you not only stimulate your mind; you also can feel more fulfilled and satisfied with your life.

Go Outside Your Box: Suggestions

Here are some suggestions on how to go outside of your comfortable zone and challenge your mind with new information that can enrich your life:

- Learn to create new recipes or cook new foods. You might take a cooking class, attend cooking demonstrations, watch cooking lessons online or on TV, or create a cooking group with others where you share and prepare new foods together.

- Learn to play a musical instrument, or return to one you learned many years ago.

- Explore a new hobby, such as painting, birdwatching, astronomy, sculpting, quilt making, calligraphy, or any of dozens of other activities. Learn on your own or with a friend—from a class, DVD, online, or book, or a combination of ways.

- Learn about a different culture, religion, or philosophy through books, DVDs, lectures, joining a group (in person or online), research online, and classes.

- Choose a historical, literary, scientific, or other person past or present who interests you and learn all you can about him or her. If you choose someone who lived in your area, you might have access to a broader wealth of information.

- Become a docent for an organization/nonprofit and be trained to help others learn more about the organization. Museums, nature centers, parks, and zoos are places that frequently train docents to help them share information about their facilities with the public.

- Go to museums and take the informational tours or lectures they offer.

- Keep up with current events and join forums where people discuss them.

- Learn about foreign places—without leaving the country! If you can travel and learn about a favorite place firsthand, that's a great learning opportunity. However, if you cannot or do not want to travel, then learn from the comfort of home. Borrow DVDs and videos from the library, go online and access travel sites, travel blogs, and Web sites about your area of interest, correspond with people who blog from your favorite locations, and borrow books on the topic. Although it's not the same as being there, it's much less expensive, and there's no jet lag!

GET OUT OF YOUR RUT

It's comforting and stabilizing to follow routines and have certain habits. Perhaps you wouldn't think of starting your day without having a cup of coffee in your favorite mug or watching the same news channel every night. But some routines can also put you into a rut and fail to challenge your brain. So take the "ruts" out of "routines" and make some of your everyday activities more challenging or mind boosting. For example:

- Get your news from more than one source: read more than one newspaper, visit different Web sites; turn to different TV stations.

- Listen to debates and/or read editorials or commentaries that explore both sides of an issue.

- If you already do crossword puzzles, do more challenging ones and break out into other word games, such as cryptograms, anagrams, and Scrabble. Do sudoku puzzles.

- Play games such as chess, checkers, Othello, and backgammon online. That way you and your virtual partner can play anytime!

- Use your head instead of a calculator to balance your checkbook, or just practice adding and multiplying numbers. For example, keep track in your mind of what you are spending while shopping for groceries.

- Don't just read a book—discuss it with others. You can join a book club or book discussion group, either in person or on the Internet.

- Don't just watch the news or read about topics that interest you—discuss them. Join a discussion group on a topic of interest, either in your community or on the Internet.

- Keep a journal or diary or write blog entries or stories. Writing strengthens the brain's ability to analyze, convey feelings and thoughts, and engage in critical thinking.

- Draw and illustrate what you write or just to have fun. Drawing stimulates the right hemisphere of the brain and stimulates creativity. Don't worry about how well you draw; just use colored pencils and express yourself.

NEUROBICS

The term "neurobics" refers to a system of brain exercises developed by Lawrence C. Katz, PhD, a professor of neurobiology at Duke University Medical Center. Several features of neurobics make it an effective, fun, and convenient way for just about anyone to stimulate their mind and sharpen their senses without the use of any special materials. And the possibilities are limited only by your imagination.

Neurobics involves using your five physical senses (smell, sight, hearing, touch, taste) and your emotional sense in ways that deviate from your normal, everyday routine. When you alter an activity that you have always done in one way, you wake up your brain and trigger underused nerve connections and pathways, thus building "brain muscle."

For example, let's say you drive the same way to work every day: you drive down your street to the highway, take the highway to exit 10, turn right, and there you are. After a while, you could probably do it with your eyes closed (figuratively, not literally!). Essentially, your brain goes to sleep every time you take that route, because nothing new is happening. Is your life full of such mindless activities?

Now it's time to shake up your brain and make some new connections. In neurobics, you take regular activities and make them new while using more than one sense if possible. For example:

- Instead of just listening to music, dance and sing along.

- Take a different route to work, the store, church, school, your friend's house.

- Use your nondominant hand to write, stir something, eat, use the TV remote, or operate your computer mouse.

- Eat with your eyes closed and concentrate on the taste and texture of the food.

- Try to identify items of clothing using touch only: keep your eyes closed while you put them on.

- Take a walk and instead of just watching the path in front of you, listen carefully for certain sounds— for example, different birdcalls, traffic, bits of conversations.

- Go to a foreign food market and explore exotic food items.

- Watch a foreign TV show and try to guess what they are saying.

- While taking a walk, try to identify as many different smells as you can.

Research indicates that people who use their nondominant hand (i.e., their left hand if they are right-handed) can help stimulate areas of their brain that they don't usually use. Thus merely using your nondominant hand for some activities can help you build up your brain. Brain exercises can be that simple!

SLEEP: THE PASSIVE BRAIN EXERCISE

Can sleep really stimulate your brain? Research indicates that sleep stimulates neurogenesis, which is the development of new nerve cells in the brain. Animal studies suggest that a lack of sufficient sleep reduces the number of new brain cells. You also need adequate sleep (seven to eight hours per night) to repair damage to brain cells, process and consolidate knowledge, and form memories. New research even suggests that fragmented or insufficient sleep can contribute to premature death among older adults.

When you sleep, the hippocampus, which is where memory is stored in the brain, is highly active, moving knowledge from short-term memory to long-term memory. The sleeping brain works with two kinds of memory. One is declarative memory, which involves information, such as names, dates, and trivia. The other is procedural memory, which is what allows you to remember how to drive, balance your checkbook, and access your e-mail.

Experts believe the consolidation of declarative memory requires slow wave sleep, while procedural memory needs rapid eye movement (REM) sleep. During slow wave sleep, also known as deep sleep or non-REM sleep, your brain waves are extremely slow and your heart and respiratory rates are very low. This is the time your body "recharges" itself: regenerating tissues, building muscle and bone, and boosting your immune system. But it is also the time when your brain solidifies your declarative memory.

Periodically during deep sleep you enter into REM sleep, when your eyes move rapidly and you experience dreams (although you may not remember them). During REM sleep your brain sorts and consolidates the day's experiences to form long-term memories. Throughout the night, you cycle between non-REM and REM sleep, and each REM cycle lasts longer than the previous one. Therefore, if you fail to get enough sleep each night, you are depriving yourself of sufficient REM sleep and thus time to form long-term memories.

Napping

Can taking a nap help your brain and memory? Yes, according to numerous studies, so you shouldn't feel guilty about taking one if you feel the need. Daytime napping can benefit declarative memory, and the advantages come from non-

REM sleep. Naps in the studies were usually ninety minutes long, which sounds like a pretty refreshing nap!

As with everything, however, there can be a downside. The most important thing to remember is to not let napping interfere with your nighttime sleep. If your naps are preventing you from getting at least a solid six to seven hours of refreshing sleep, then it may be time to readjust your sleeping patterns.

Reasons to consider napping are: (1) if you want to make planned naps part of your everyday routine; (2) if you are experiencing unexpected tiredness or sleepiness; or (3) if you know you are going to lose sleep because of a long work shift, travel arrangements, or another reason.

When it comes to suggestions on the best way to take a nap, the recommendations vary widely. Some experts say to nap for only ten to thirty minutes, noting that the longer your nap the mort likely you will wake up feeling groggy. The length of your nap is something with which you will need to experiment. You can reap some brain benefits from a thirty-minute nap, but you are more likely to help your memory with a longer nap. However, if you find that a longer nap has a negative impact on your ability to function for the rest of the day, then that long nap is probably not helping you. Also, not everyone has the luxury of free time to take a long nap.

The best time for a nap is usually between 2 and 3 PM, a time that is least likely to interfere with nighttime sleep. Your lifestyle may prevent you from claiming this time as nap time, however, if you work, but the weekends may give you a chance to catch up on missed sleep and brain-boosting time!

HIGH-TECH BRAIN BOOSTERS

Computers, the Internet, DVDs, and video games have opened doors to fun, interesting, and convenient ways for people to challenge and stimulate their brain. Even if you don't own a computer, most public libraries allow access to their computers if you have a library card.

Scores of brain-boosting games and exercises are available on these free venues, whether you access them from home or a Wi-Fi spot. (See box below.) These games and exercises can provide you with hours of stimulating fun, and you can use them any hour of the day or night.

BRAIN GAMES ON THE INTERNET

Some Web sites have free (or mostly free) brain games you can access and play anytime. These Web sites are offered as possibilities only; access and rules of use may change at any time. You can also explore the Internet for many more possibilities.

http://playwithyourmind.com/
http://www.mybraintrainer.com/
http://www.freebrainagegames.com/
http://www.braintraining101.com/
http://www.brainmetrix.com/
http://www.braingle.com/
http://www.sharpbrains.com/teasers/brain-games-and-teasers-top-50/
http://www.brainpractices.com/
http://www.realage.com/ (Search for brain games.)
http://www.zynga.com/

MANAGE STRESS TO BOOST BRAINPOWER

Managing stress is so important for fighting aging that an entire chapter is devoted to it. However, I want to mention it here so you realize just how critical proper stress management is if you want to preserve and maintain your brain health.

The impact of stress on the brain is significant. In fact, stress can cause atrophy (shrinkage) of the hippocampus, an area of the brain critical for episodic, spatial, and contextual memory. If you experience stress that is severe and lasts for weeks or months, it can hinder cell communication in your brain and have a negative impact on your ability to learn and remember.

Even short-term stress can be damaging. University of California researchers found that stress lasting just a few hours can hamper brain-cell communication in areas of the brain involved with memory and learning. More specifically, short-term stress activates molecules called corticotropin-releasing hormones, which interfere with the process involved in collecting and storing memories in the brain.

So, if you want to help maintain good brain health, make sure you manage your stress. You can find many suggestions in Step 9.

LAUGHTER IMPROVES MEMORY

It's definitely a laughing matter: the giggles are good for your brain. Not only can laughter help you think better; it can also increase your memory capacity and enhance your ability to focus and concentrate.

When you laugh, there's much more going on behind the look of amusement or happiness on your face. Scientists have verified the healing power of humor through numerous studies. When you laugh and have fun, your stress levels decline. Laughter reduces the production of hormones associated with stress, which disrupt the function of the immune system. When you laugh, your body produces more cells that fight disease, called gamma-interferon T cells. Laughter also stimulates the areas of the brain that use dopamine, the "feel good" chemical messenger.

Scientists have studied the impact of humor and laughter on longevity. In a study from the University of Akron (Ohio), investigators found that thirty-three older adults who rated themselves and a deceased sibling on a humor scale found a significant difference between the appreciation of humor and longevity in the surviving sibling and the sibling who had died.

Perhaps doctors should prescribe laughter, write a prescription for it to be enjoyed at least several times a day in hearty doses. Because laughter is such a great stress reducer, it is discussed in Step 9 as part of stress management.

So make sure to take time out each day to laugh: read some jokes, watch a TV show or movie that makes you laugh, look at funny videos on YouTube or others on the Internet, or call a friend who makes you laugh. What if you can't find anything that tickles your funny bone? Maybe you need a laughter coach. Don't laugh (or do laugh!); it's true. There are laughter coaches who teach people to laugh "effectively," as well as laughter clubs that have popped up around the world. The idea is that laughter is a social phenomenon and thus contagious. If you hear someone laugh, the laughter releases a neurotransmitter in your brain that in turn releases chemicals in the body. Thus laughter, like a yawn, is "catching." And considering the benefits of laughter, there are much worse things you could catch.

FEED YOUR BRAIN

If you read Step 1—and I hope you did!—you know how critical it is to choose the best possible food if you want to achieve and maintain good health and add vital years to your life. But those foods don't only nourish your body—they are also necessary for optimal brain functioning. Because certain foods are especially important for brain health, I will mention them again here—but that's no excuse not to thoroughly devour Step 1.

- Omega-3 fatty acids are found mainly in cold-water fish (e.g., salmon, herring, halibut, tuna) as well as flaxseed and walnuts. These fatty acids are necessary for the structural and functional integrity of the brain. Of the two main omega-3s, docosahexaenoic acid (DHA) and eicosapentaenoic acid (EPA), DHA makes up much of the gray matter in the brain and is necessary for brain cell function and communication. A diet rich in DHA can improve learning, while a deficiency can worsen your ability to retain new material. (Read more about omega-3s in Step 6.)

- Vegetables are excellent sources of antioxidants, which fight brain-cell-damaging free radicals. Research also suggests eating vegetables helps slow mental decline.

- Foods rich in the B vitamins folic acid, B_6, and B_{12} are important for the brain because they help lower your levels of homocysteine, a nonprotein amino acid that is a strong risk factor for dementia. Whole grains and leafy green vegetables are good sources of B vitamins.

- A moderate amount of red wine per day may protect your brain cells because this beverage contains resveratrol, a polyphenol that has potent antioxidant properties and an ability to protect brain cells. (See Step 6.) However, if you don't already drink, this is not an invitation to start!

- Blueberries and other foods rich in flavonoids, especially anthocyanins and flavanols, have been shown to improve short-term memory loss and even reverse age-related brain decline. So far scientists aren't sure exactly how these plant-derived substances affect the brain, but one theory is that they boost existing connections between neurons, improve communication between cells, and stimulate regeneration of neurons. Raspberries, cherries, purple grapes, and red cabbage are also excellent sources of anthocyanins.

EXERCISE YOUR BODY, ENHANCE YOUR BRAIN

Here is another example of the intimate connection between the mind and body. Because physical exercise is discussed in detail in Step 3, I mention it again here only to highlight its importance in promoting a younger, healthier brain. Exercise boosts brain function by stimulating the formation of new brain cells as well as the connections between them. Physical exercise can also stimulate areas of the brain that are associated with learning and memory. And in the fight against the possibility of Alzheimer's disease scientists have found that exercise reduces the risk of cognitive decline and dementia in older adults.

So make sure you don't skip Step 3, because if you don't you'll be doing both your body and your brain a big favor!

SOCIALIZE FOR A BETTER BRAIN

Socializing with other people is a form of mental exercise, and therefore it can help keep your brain sharp. Social interaction can take various forms: talking on the phone or on Skype, sending e-mails, meeting in person with family and friends, interacting with coworkers, and attending events or venues where there is some personal interaction, such as school, church, clubs, parties, and meetings.

The impact of socializing on brain health and memory has been studied relatively well, and the hands-down consensus is that social ties are critical for both mental and physical health. In fact, having no social ties is believed to be a risk factor for mental decline in older adults. In a Harvard study of more than twenty-eight hundred people age 65 and older, those who had at least five social ties—phone callers, regular visitors, social groups, church groups, et cetera—were less likely to experience a decline in cognition than those who had no social ties. Another study found that talking to another person for just ten minutes a day can improve memory and test scores and that socializing can boost memory and intellectual performance.

Many more benefits of socializing on helping you stay younger, healthier, and smarter and numerous ways to broaden your social interactions are covered in Step 7.

DRUGS THAT MAY DAMAGE YOUR MEMORY

One part of keeping your brain healthy and functioning at its best is understanding what factors can harm it and jeopardize your attempts to keep your mind operating at its best. Common and often-overlooked memory manipulators are medications, especially prescriptions. Some medications (called anticholinergics) block the activity of a critical brain chemical called acetylcholine, and lowered levels of this chemical can impair your mental function, especially as you get older. If you are taking any of the following medications or if you suspect something else you are taking may be affecting your memory, talk to your doctor about switching to another drug.

Antidiarrhea drugs

- Atrophine-diphenoxylate (Lomotil, Lonox)

- Genitourinary drugs (e.g., antibiotics for urinary tract infections such as amoxicillin, cefazolin)

- Oxybutynin (Ditropan)

- Perphenazine

Antihistamines/Sleep Aids

- Chlorpheniramine (Allerest)

- Cyproheptadine (Periactin)

- Diphenhydramine (Benadryl, Sominex, Unisom, others)

- Hydroxyzine (Atarax, Vistaril)

- Promethazine (Phenergan)

Antihypertensives

- Nifedipine (Adalat, Procardia)

Antipsychotics

- Chlorpromazine (Thorazine)

- Haloperidol (Haldol)

- Thioridazine (Mellaril)

Antispasmodics

- Darifenacin (Enablex)

- Dicyclomine (Bentyl)

- Fesoterodine (Toviaz)

- Hyoscyamine (Anaspaz, Levbid, Levsin, others)

- Tolterodine (Detrol)

Bronchodilators

- Ipratropium bromide (Atrovent)
- Tiotropium (SPIRIVA)

Histamine-2 Blockers

- Cimetidine (Tagamet)
- Famotidine (Pepcid)
- Ranitidine (Zantac)

Muscle Relaxants

- Carisoprodol (Soma)
- Cyclobenzaprine (Flexeril)
- Metaxalone (Skelaxin)
- Methocarbamol (Robaxin)

Antidepressants

- Amitriptyline (Elavil)
- Desipramine (Norpramin)
- Doxepin (Sinequan)
- Imipramine (Tofranil)
- Nortriptyline (Pamelor)
- Venlafaxine XR (EFFEXOR XR)

STEP 6

Choose Supplements Every Body Needs

If you listen to some antiaging commercials and ads, you might think you need to take dozens of supplements and spend hundreds of dollars a month to help stay young, vital, and mentally sharp. Yet if you follow the other nine steps outlined in this book, your need for supplements could be minimal. The one thing many people forget about supplements is what they are: *supplements,* not replacements for nutritious food and healthy lifestyle habits. Popping a multivitamin and calcium supplement every day won't make up for a diet consisting of fast-food burgers and pizza and unmanaged stress. What well-chosen supplements can do, however, is support your other age-defying efforts to maintain your physical and emotional/mental health as your body undergoes the many changes associated with aging.

One bit of good news is that research into the benefits of natural supplements is vigorous, so there are new findings coming out all the time. Keeping up with the ongoing research is exciting, and I urge you to follow the developments of supplements as they make the news. To get you started, this chapter offers details on ten supplements from which every aging body can benefit: alpha lipoic acid, B complex, betaine, calcium, coenzyme Q10, green tea, omega-3 fatty acids, pterostilbene, resveratrol, and vitamin D. You may choose to take one or more of these supplements; the choice will be up to you. (Always consult a knowledgeable health-care professional before starting any supplement program.)

ALPHA LIPOIC ACID

Alpha lipoic acid (ALA) is a vitamin-like substance that has potent antioxidant properties. ALA is found in small amounts in most foods, although spinach and other green leafy vegetables, yeast, broccoli, liver, and potatoes deliver higher levels.

Your body needs ALA to produce energy, and the nutrient has an important role in the energy-producing organelles in cells. Although the body can produce a sufficient amount of ALA for these purposes, its antioxidant powers kick in when your body has an excess of ALA and it exists in a "free" state in your cells. Since your body typically has little free ALA, that's where a supplement can come in handy when you want to challenge the aging process.

Alpha Lipoic Acid, Health, and Aging

Why is alpha lipoic acid viewed as an antiaging supplement? A number of research studies have provided some potential and convincing reasons.

- Alpha lipoic acid is capable of passing into the brain—a feat not many nutrients can claim—where it helps regenerate other antioxidants, such as vitamins C and E, and glutathione, the "master" antioxidant. Glutathione can't be taken directly as an oral supplement because the body metabolizes it, so alpha lipoic acid is the next best way to get this critical antioxidant. (Read more about glutathione later.)

- ALA is a chelator, which means it has the ability to attract toxic metals such as aluminum, lead, mercury, and cadmium—all of which generate cell-damaging free radicals—and remove them from the body. This is important for obvious reasons but also because the removal of heavy metals may help in the prevention of Alzheimer's disease.

- Alpha lipoic acid is both water and fat soluble, which makes it easily absorbed from your gut.

- For people with diabetes, alpha lipoic acid can help manage the nerve-related symptoms of the disease, such as burning, pain, and numbness in the arms and legs.

- ALA can reduce fasting blood glucose and insulin resistance if you have type 2 diabetes and help manage blood sugar levels. These are especially important characteristics because uncontrolled blood sugar levels can accelerate the aging process.

- Alpha lipoic acid has anti-inflammatory abilities, which are important for prevention of heart disease, arthritis, and other age-related conditions associated with inflammation.

- Eye-related conditions such as glaucoma, cataracts, and Wilson's disease can benefit from alpha lipoic acid supplementation.

- Animal studies suggest alpha lipoic acid supplementation may help with memory and oxidative stress.

Scores of animal studies indicate that ALA has an ability to slow down the aging process, improve blood circulation, enhance the immune system, and benefit other bodily functions as well. How does it accomplish these things? Using animal models, researchers at Oregon State University discovered that alpha lipoic acid turns on basic cellular defenses, including some of those that naturally decline as you get older, and helps cells recover their functions.

Alpha Lipoic Acid and Glutathione

A special characteristic of ALA is its ability to help restore glutathione levels to near normal. Glutathione is a critical nutrient for many reasons. (See "Glutathione: The Great Antioxidant" below.) For example, glutathione assists the liver in removing foreign chemicals from the body, including pollutants, heavy metals, and drugs—substances that can contribute to aging. Glutathione is intimately involved with protein synthesis, protection of the mitochondria (the cell's energy production organelle) and cell membranes, metabolism, and maturation of your cells.

However, taking glutathione as a supplement is a problem, because the body will break it down unless you take it as an injection. Therefore, ALA supplementation serves as a catalyst to boost glutathione levels.

GLUTATHIONE: THE GREAT ANTIOXIDANT

If you are considering taking ALA, here are some comments by experts concerning the importance of glutathione as an age-defying supplement:

- Earl Mindell, RPH, MH, PhD, author of *Earl Mindell's Vitamin Bible, Dr. Earl Mindell's What You Should Know about the Super Antioxidant Miracle,* and dozens of other books, says: "We literally cannot survive without this miraculous antioxidant."

- Jimmy Gutman, MD, FACEP, and author of *Glutathione: Essential Health AID—Antioxidant. Immune Booster. Detoxifier,* wrote: "Healthy people also benefit from elevated glutathione levels through an enhanced ability to fight off toxins, infectious disease, precancerous cells and the aging process itself." He also states that glutathione levels decline as people age and that "many diseases normally associated with aging have been linked to glutathione deficiency."

- Lorna R. Vanderhaeghe and Patrick J. D. Bouic, PhD, in *The Immune System Cure,* note: "No other antioxidant is as important to overall health as glutathione. . . . Low levels are associated with early aging and even death."

- A study published by Julius M. et al. in the *Journal of Clinical Epidemiology* notes: "Lower glutathione levels are implicated in many diseases associated with aging, including cataracts, Alzheimer's disease, Parkinson's, atherosclerosis and others."

How to Take Alpha Lipoic Acid

Alpha lipoic acid is available as capsules. Your health-care provider can also give you an injection if you prefer. No specific dose for ALA has been established, although a general recommendation is 20 to 80 milligrams daily for support of the immune system. People with diabetes and diabetic neuropathy may take up to 800 milligrams daily in divided doses, but naturally you should first check with your doctor.

If you have diabetes, talk to your health-care provider before taking ALA, because it can combine with any diabetes medications you may be taking and cause your blood sugar levels to drop too low (hypoglycemia). Also, if you are taking any thyroid medication, ALA may reduce your thyroid hormone levels. You and your health-care provider should watch your thyroid function tests. Side effects associated with ALA are relatively rare and may include rash.

B COMPLEX

A B-complex supplement is typically defined as a product that supplies thiamine (B_1), riboflavin (B_2), niacin (B_3), pantothenic acid (B_5), pyridoxine (B_6), biotin, folic acid, the cobalamins (B_{12}), choline, inositol, and sometimes para-aminobenzoic acid (PABA), a vitamin-like substance that is not "officially" a B vitamin. Each B vitamin has a unique structure and tasks, but because it is a family each element works in conjunction with the other members in some fashion. Although not all experts agree, many say it is best to take all the B vitamins in combination rather than individually, unless you have been instructed to take a specific dose of one or more of the B vitamins for a certain reason.

Generally, some of the B vitamins help your cells burn sugars and fats for energy, assist in the production of neurotransmitters (chemicals that are necessary for healthy brain function), promote cell growth and division (including your red blood cells), and maintain healthy muscle tone, hair, and skin. But some of the B vitamins are especially important when it comes to aging.

B Vitamins, Health, and Aging

The B vitamins provide a number of health and antiaging benefits. One is their ability to promote a calmer mood and thus help reduce stress and its aging consequences. Perhaps the most well-known benefit associated with B vitamins is the ability of three of them—folic acid, B_6, and B_{12}—to help lower levels of homocysteine, an amino acid associated with an increased risk of heart disease. It's been shown that people who have high homocysteine levels are thirty times more likely to develop vascular disease than individuals who have normal levels. That makes homocysteine an even more important risk factor for heart disease than high cholesterol, smoking cigarettes, or high blood pressure. Sounds like these

B vitamins are important when it comes to fighting a disease so common among aging adults!

Here's another reason to take B vitamins: high levels of homocysteine are associated with aging features—brain shrinkage, cognitive impairment, and dementia. In a two-year Oxford study, 168 individuals were given either a megadose of B vitamins or a placebo. The brains of people in the vitamin group shrank only 0.76 percent per year while those in the placebo group shrank 1.08 percent per year, for a difference of 53 percent. In addition, the people in the vitamin group performed better on cognitive tests and the individuals who had the most significant slowing of atrophy were the ones who had the highest homocysteine levels at the beginning of the study.

In addition to B_6, B_{12}, and folic acid and their role in lowering homocysteine level, these and other B vitamins have other roles in helping you defy aging and its consequences. For example:

- Vitamin B_3 is involved in repairing DNA, a critical function in the fight against aging and cancer.

- Pantothenic acid is involved in reducing cholesterol levels and can speed up your recovery from wounds, including surgery.

- Folic acid may lower your risk of stroke and colon cancer.

- Biotin plus chromium (a mineral) improves control of blood sugar.

- Vitamin B_{12} can help with memory and mental "fog."

- Choline is necessary for normal brain and memory function.

- PABA assists with the production of folic acid in the intestinal tract. You may also recognize PABA as an ingredient in some sunscreens, and that's because it can protect your skin against ultraviolet radiation.

How to Take B-Complex Supplements

The best food sources of B vitamins include dark green leafy vegetables, whole grains, and nuts and seeds. If you don't get enough B vitamins from your diet, you may want to take a B-complex supplement.

Take a B-complex supplement early in the day and with food, because it has been known to cause nausea if you take it on an empty stomach. The vitamin B_6 component can cause an increase in disruptive dreaming if you take it late in the day.

When choosing a B-complex supplement, look for those that contain the level of B vitamins recommended by your health-care professional, because the levels of vitamins can vary greatly. The dosage selected by your physician should take into account your diet, stress level, and health issues. Therefore, if you are experiencing chronic stress or anxiety you may need to take a higher level of B vitamins than if you are in generally good health and following a healthy diet.

For example:

- If you are in good health and younger than 30, a low-potency B-complex supplement is likely sufficient. If you are also taking a multivitamin, check the label, as you may already be taking enough of the B vitamins.

- Even if you eat foods rich in B vitamins, if you take one or more over-the-counter or prescription medications (e.g., those for reflux disease, heartburn, and high blood pressure, as well as diuretics, oral antibiotics, and contraceptives) you may need to take a B-complex because these drugs can interfere with the absorption of certain B vitamins.

- Use of alcohol depletes several B vitamins, especially B_1 and B_3, so if alcohol is a regular part of your lifestyle you should consider taking a moderate-level B-complex supplement.

BETAINE (TRIMETHYLGLYCINE)

Betaine, also referred to as trimethylglycine (TMG), is a nutritional component found in small quantities in some plant foods, including broccoli, whole grains, beets, and spinach. The human body can manufacture betaine from choline, so if your diet is low in betaine your body will likely maintain a healthy level of the nutrient. However, it you take a betaine supplement, you "free up" some choline for its other tasks, such as making acetylcholine and phosphatidylcholine, substances that are important for memory and brain function.

Betaine, Health, and Aging

Betaine is considered to be one of the more important antiaging nutrients, and one reason is because it is a methyl donor that helps in the process of methylation. This means that betaine donates a portion of itself—a methyl group composed of a carbon atom attached to three hydrogen atoms—to another substance so a chemical modification process called methylation can occur. Betaine is a critical part of the methylation process that reduces levels of homocysteine, an amino acid that has been linked to an increased risk of heart disease, stroke, heart attack, Alzheimer's disease, and Parkinson's disease. Because the body's ability to methylate appears to decline with age, thus contributing to the aging process, supplementation may be a way to resist aging.

Betaine is also associated with other age-defying benefits:

- Betaine can reduce levels of C-reactive protein, a substance associated with inflammation.

- Sufficient methylation of DNA can prevent the expression of cancer genes; thus betaine may support and promote adequate methylation and help ward off cancer.

- As a methyl donor, betaine assists in the production of brain chemicals that are involved with mood, energy, alertness, and concentration.

- During aging, betaine suppresses certain inflammatory factors, such as NF-kappaB, which controls inflammatory molecules involved in cancer, atherosclerosis, and arthritis.

- Betaine may also protect nerve fibers and improve symptoms of Parkinson's disease and Alzheimer's disease.

- Betaine protects the liver against damage from alcohol.

- The DNA protection properties of betaine may slow the progression of cell aging.

How to Take Betaine Supplements

Betaine supplements are available as capsules, tablets, and a powder and are made as a by-product of sugar-beet processing. No optimal dose of betaine has been established thus far, although a typical dosage is 375 to 1,000 milligrams daily. Use of vitamins B_6, B_{12}, and folic acid enhance the benefits of betaine. Side effects have not been reported. If you have kidney or liver disease, talk to your doctor before taking betaine.

CALCIUM

Calcium is the most abundant mineral in the human body and the one nutrient most often associated with bones. Do you remember your mother or father telling you to drink your milk so you would build strong bones? Well, you're older now, but calcium is still an essential nutrient for bone health, and much more, as you age.

Calcium and Your Aging Brain

One of the lesser-known facts about calcium is that it is essential for healthy brain function. For example, when a chemical signal makes contact with a brain cell (neuron) it needs help to get inside the cell. That's the job of calcium ions: to deliver signals to the inside of cells. Healthy brain cells require a specific amount of calcium, and if that level gets too high a complex pumping system composed of proteins moves the excess calcium out of the cell. If the pump system fails, too much calcium will build up and kill the brain cell.

The hitch in this system is that as you age the proteins that make up the pumping system disappear from older brain cells, and the cells that still have pumps are not as effective as they were when you were younger. This combination of events means calcium levels within the cells can build up and stress, even kill, your brain cells.

To keep those pump proteins active, researchers have found that reducing calorie intake, which in turn reduces the production of free radicals, can help maintain a healthy calcium balance in your brain and also reduce cell death. Other ways to protect the proteins include the following:

- Take red Korean ginseng, which has been shown to moderate the activity of the pumps.

- Take vitamin D, which can reduce the effect of age-related processes in brain cells.

- Consume lots of antioxidants in the form of food (especially fruits and vegetables) and supplements, such as grape seed and other berry extracts, coenzyme Q10, and green tea (both of which are discussed in this chapter), and lipoic acid, can help maintain the energy producers in your brain cells.

Calcium and Aging

Ninety-nine percent of the calcium in your body is stored in your bones and teeth. Your bones undergo continuous resorption and deposition of calcium, and these processes change as you age. During your bone-building years, your body absorbed as much as 60 percent of the calcium you consumed in food and supplements. That absorption rate declined dramatically to 15 percent and to 20 percent when you reached adulthood, and it keeps on declining as you get older, with the breakdown of bone exceeding bone formation. The result can be osteoporosis and the possibility of fractures, both of which you want to avoid. To do that, you want to make sure you get enough calcium—but not too much. Here's the story.

Calcium: How Much Do You Need?

The latest report from the Institute of Medicine (2011), which periodically reviews and updates the Dietary Reference Intakes (DRIs), recommends 1,000 milligrams daily for all adults ages 19 through 50 and for men until age 71. The daily recommendation goes up to 1,200 milligrams daily beginning at age 51 for women and at age 71 for men. Higher amounts are not necessary for bone health, overall health, or longevity and, in fact, can be detrimental. Therefore, not everyone needs to take calcium supplements.

If you get much of your calcium from supplements, for example, you increase your risk of developing kidney stones. Among men, there is growing evidence that too much calcium is a risk factor for prostate cancer. Too much calcium can also cause constipation and may interfere with the absorption of zinc and iron. Therefore, to be safe take into account the amount of calcium you get from your diet and do not take more of a calcium supplement than you need.

If you do take a calcium supplement, you should know that the efficiency of absorption decreases as your intake of calcium increases, so you don't want to take a large dose of the supplement at one time—500 milligrams is the maximum dose. Finally, calcium is best absorbed if your body has a sufficient amount of vitamin D. You can read more about vitamin D in this chapter.

How to Take Calcium Supplements

Which type of calcium supplement is best? This is one of the most often asked questions among people who want to take a calcium supplement. Although there are about half a dozen different types, the final decision is usually between calcium carbonate and calcium citrate. Calcium carbonate is the form found in about 85 percent of calcium supplements in the United States, and it also usually less expensive than all the other forms. The supplement should be taken twice daily with food for optimal absorption, preferably at breakfast and dinner.

Compared with calcium citrate, the carbonate form has about twice the amount of elemental calcium by weight. This means you need to take fewer or smaller tablets to get the recommended amount of elemental calcium, which is the calcium your body actually uses. So, if you take a 1,000 milligram tablet of calcium carbonate, 400 milligrams (40 percent) of the tablet is elemental calcium. The recommended dose refers to the amount of elemental calcium; therefore, the % DV (daily value) of 100 percent is equal to 1,000 milligrams of elemental calcium.

You can take either calcium carbonate or calcium citrate with acid-reducing medications such as antacids and prescriptions such as Prilosec. They are also appropriate if you have heartburn, gastroesophageal reflux disease (GERD), achlorhydria, and hypochlorhydria (lack of stomach acid and too little stomach acid, respectively).

COENZYME Q10

Coenzyme Q10 (CoQ10) is a substance that can be found in nearly every cell in your body, which is a strong indication of its importance. As a potent antioxidant, CoQ10 can fight free radicals that contribute to the aging process, as well as perform its other major task: assisting in the conversion of food into energy.

The main food sources of CoQ10 include whole grains, oily fish (e.g., tuna, salmon), and organ meats (e.g., liver). While a well-balanced diet can provide an adequate amount of CoQ10, adding a supplement to your routine as you age may be to your advantage.

CoQ10, Health, and Aging

Experts know that CoQ10 levels decline as you age and that smoking also contributes to its loss. While levels are highest during the first two decades of your life, they can fall to below what they were at birth by the time you are 80. So if late in life you were to take CoQ10 supplements to raise your levels to your age-20 range, could you extend your life? Thus far, scientists have not found this to be true in any organisms except bacteria, although at least one study did find that CoQ10 supplementation reduced the age-related increase in DNA damage.

One area where experts have found convincing evidence of some age-defying benefits of CoQ10 is heart health, which is why some doctors prescribe the supplement for individuals who have heart- and blood vessel–related conditions. For example:

- CoQ10 taken after a heart attack can reduce the likelihood of a subsequent attack and chest pain.

- Studies also suggest that people with heart failure who take CoQ10 along with conventional medications experience improved breathing, less swelling in their legs, reduced fluid in their lungs, and better exercise capacity.

- Blood pressure (BP) typically rises as you age, and CoQ10 has been shown to lower both systolic (the upper number of a BP reading) and diastolic pressures, although it may take four to twelve weeks before you see a significant change.

- If high cholesterol is an issue for you and you are taking statin drugs, CoQ10 can help. Statins reduce your body's natural levels of CoQ10, so taking a supplement can help restore your levels, as well as reduce muscle pain associated with statin use.

- CoQ10 supplements may improve hemoglobin A1c levels (a measure of long-term control of blood sugar) in people who have diabetes.

- If you are scheduled for heart surgery, taking CoQ10 before your procedure can reduce free-radical damage, reduce the incidence of irregular heartbeats during your recovery, and strengthen heart function.

How to Take CoQ10 Supplements

CoQ10 supplements are available as hard-shell capsules, softgel capsules, tablets, and an oral spray. The recommended dose for adults is 30 to 200 milligrams daily, depending on the reason your doctor has agreed you can take this supplement. The body tends to absorb the soft gels better than the other forms, and for maximum absorption take the supplement with a meal that contains some fat. If you take more than one dose per day, make sure one of those doses is at dinner, because CoQ10 seems to be better utilized at night.

Coenzyme Q10 is generally safe and associated with no major side effects, although some people experience mild stomach upset. If you have diabetes, definitely talk to your doctor before taking the supplement, because it may lower your blood sugar too far.

GREEN TEA

Since ancient times, green tea has been valued both as a beverage and for its medicinal properties. Like all true teas—which should not be confused with flower and herbal infusions that are commonly called teas—green tea comes from the *Camellia sinensis* plant. What makes green tea different from oolong and black teas is how it's made: the fresh leaves are steamed at high temperatures but are not fermented (oxidized), whereas the leaves used to make oolong and black teas are. This minimal processing allows green tea leaves to retain their high antioxidant properties and, along with them, a greater ability to fight free radicals and aging.

Enjoying several cups of green tea each day—as noted in Step 1—is one way to take advantage of the antioxidants, but green tea supplements are also available if you want to boost the power of the beverage or if this brew is just not, well, your cup of tea.

Green Tea, Health, and Aging

In recent years researchers have been providing scientific evidence to back up the claims made over the millennia about the medicinal value of green tea. Experts now know that credit for green tea's benefits, including antiaging, goes to antioxidants called polyphenols. In particular, antioxidants in a category called catechins are believed to play a pivotal role in green tea's health-promoting abilities, with special emphasis on one called epigallocatechin-3-gallate (EGCG).

One age-defying property of EGCG appears to be its ability to inhibit telomere shortening, especially related to

heart dysfunction. Here are a few other age-defying benefits attributed to green tea, EGCG, and some of its other
constituents:

- Green tea can lower glucose levels, which is an important antiaging benefit. One study of both green
  and black teas found that green tea lowered blood
  sugar slightly better than black tea, but it was much
  better at reducing triglycerides, which are associated with a high risk of cardiovascular disease.

- Green tea also has another sugar-lowering ingredient called diphenylamine. Along with EGCG, these
  two compounds—and there may be more as scientists continue their research—can help manage
  blood sugar levels.

- Green tea may help you drop excess pounds. A
  number of studies support this claim, although the
  exact reason for this benefit isn't clear. One may be
  the ability of green tea to reduce the release and
  absorption of glucose, which helps control weight.
  The caffeine in green tea may boost metabolism,
  although the amount of this stimulant is low in green
  tea. Yet another possibility is that high amounts of
  catechins have been shown to increase excretion of
  fat in animals. If this is also true for people, greater
  fat elimination could be another way green tea may
  help with weight loss.

- Green tea reduces the absorption of iron, which is an
  antiaging benefit.

- The health of your heart and blood vessels can be
  enhanced by green tea. In addition to lowering
  total cholesterol and low-density lipoprotein (LDL)
  cholesterol, green tea also raises high-density lipoprotein (HDL) cholesterol.

- The catechins in green tea can inhibit the proliferation of smooth muscle cells, which line the blood vessels. Such rapid growth of smooth muscle cells is a significant factor in heart disease and atherosclerosis.

- Polyphenols in green tea may prevent swelling and inflammation, protect cartilage between your bones, and reduce wear and tear on your joints, all of which are important in arthritis.

- The small amount of caffeine in green tea may help with alertness and mental function, as well as increase the release of neurotransmitters in the brain.

- The ability of green tea to prevent or manage various types of cancer is an area of much investigation, and thus far the study results are mixed: some report a small to substantial benefit (e.g., for bladder cancer) from green tea while others show no benefit or even a slightly increased risk, as with stomach cancer. Much more research is necessary around the question of the role of green tea in preventing or managing cancer.

- Let's not forget the effect of green tea on the brain, where the catechins may be helpful in preventing death of neurons. The flavonoids in general can regulate levels of nitric oxide in the brain, which is helpful because abnormally high amounts of nitric oxide can result in the death of brain cells.

How to Take Green Tea Supplements

Feel free to drink green tea along with taking the supplements (after checking with your doctor). One cup of green tea provides 20 to 35 milligrams of EGCG and about ten times more polyphenols overall. Studies suggest health advantages from green tea can be expected from consuming anywhere from 240 to 500 milligrams or more of polyphenols daily. Look for green tea supplements that list the percentage and amount of EGCG and polyphenols in each dose. Unless you like to drink lots of green tea, you might include a green tea supplement daily to increase your intake of its potent antioxidants as part of your daily routine.

Some people experience insomnia, irritability, and dizziness if they take excessive amounts of green tea extract or drink too much green tea, and this is associated with the caffeine. Decaffeinated green tea supplements and loose tea are also available if you should have any side effects. Also, talk to your doctor if you have heart problems or a kidney disorder, stomach ulcers, or an anxiety disorder, as then green tea supplements are likely best avoided or can be taken in low doses.

OMEGA-3 FATTY ACIDS

Omega-3 fatty acids are essential fatty acids, which means your body requires them to function optimally, but you are not able to produce them. Thus food and supplements are the only ways to get the omega-3s your body needs.

Of the three main omega-3 fatty acids (eicosapentaenoic acid [EPA], docosahexaenoic acid [DHA], and ALA), your body can readily utilize the former two once you consume them, but your body must first convert ALA to EPA and DHA for it to be beneficial. The main food sources of EPA and DHA are fatty fish, such as tuna, salmon, herring, halibut, and mackerel, while algae oil provides DHA only. Plants like flax and walnuts contain ALA.

Unfortunately, most people do not get enough omega-3s in their diet, and a common excuse is, "I don't like fish," or, "Fish is okay, but I just don't eat it very often." If you *really* can't include enough omega-3-rich fish in your life, then supplements are an alternative.

Omega-3s, Health, and Aging

The health benefits of omega-3s are a topic of much research, and the findings thus far have been promising as well as helpful for many people. Here's some of what you might expect from taking omega-3 fatty acids:

- Omega-3s are perhaps best known for their anti-inflammatory ability, and since inflammation is implicated in many age-related conditions this property makes omega-3s especially important. Much of the good news concerning omega-3s is in the areas of brain, heart, and blood vessel health. In fact, although both EPA and DHA are important for brain function, the highest-functioning areas of the brain contain extremely high levels of DHA, so it's important to maintain sufficient levels of this nutrient for optimal brain function.

- Fish oil supplements, which are the main type of omega-3 supplement, have been shown to significantly reduce triglyceride levels. A diet that contains several servings per week of omega-3-rich fish can increase HDL cholesterol (the good cholesterol) and lower triglycerides.

- The aging effects of high blood pressure may be alleviated with omega-3 supplements. A mega-analysis of seventeen clinical studies found that taking 3 grams or more of fish oil supplements daily lowered blood pressure in patients, even those who had untreated hypertension.

- A Harvard Medical School and Brigham and Women's Hospital literature review (November 2011) revealed the benefits of omega-3 fatty acids are consistent for preventing coronary heart disease and sudden cardiac death and also beneficial (but less established) for stroke, heart failure, heart attack, and atrial fibrillation.

- Omega-3s can boost the amount of calcium in your body and thus improve your bone health. A lack of sufficient omega-3s can lead to more bone loss when compared with regular intake of these fatty acids, according to several studies.

- Macular degeneration, a leading cause of vision loss and blindness among people age 60 and older, is less likely to develop among people who consume a diet rich in fish.

- If you've heard the saying "fish is brain food," there is some truth to it. Low intake of omega-3 fatty acids can put individuals at greater risk of developing cognitive problems, dementia, and Alzheimer's disease, and so it stands to reason that increasing your intake of omega-3s would benefit your brain. Now scientists are setting out to prove (or disprove) this hypothesis, and so far limited research indicates that DHA has a positive impact on cognitive decline.

- Understanding the role of omega-3s in preventing or managing various cancers is still in its infancy, but many studies indicate that maintaining an omega-3-rich diet and/or supplementation program can protect you from some cancers, including colorectal cancer, breast cancer, and prostate cancer.

Omega-3 and Omega-6: The Need for Balance

The "other" essential fatty acid is omega-6, and unlike its cousin, most people consume way too much omega-6 in foods such as oils, meats, and processed foods. An imbalance of the two essential fatty acids in which omega-6s are too plentiful is believed by many experts to be the cause or contributing factor in many chronic diseases, and here's one reason why.

According to Andrew Weil, MD, the internationally known complementary-medicine physician, the body makes hormones from both omega-3 and omega-6 fatty acids. Generally (but not always), the hormones from omega-6 fatty acids cause inflammation, cell proliferation, and blood clotting, while those made from omega-3 fatty acids reduce all of these activities. Since inflammation, in particular, is associated with heart disease, aging, some cancers, neurodegenerative diseases, arthritis, and other health challenges, tipping the scale in favor of omega-6 fatty acids is not a healthy situation. Therefore, to achieve a healthy balance of omega-3 and omega-6, you will likely need to take an omega-3 supplement while also reducing intake of omega-6s in your diet.

How to Take Omega-3 Fatty Acids

If eating at least two servings of cold-water fatty fish per week is not part of your menu, then it's time to turn to a fish oil supplement. Although there is no recommended standard dose of omega-3, several health-related organizations have weighed in on their suggestions. The American Heart Association, for example, recommends taking 1 gram of EPA and DHA daily if you have a heart condition and two to four times that amount if your goal is to lower your triglyceride levels and 3 to 4 grams if you have high blood pressure. If you are otherwise healthy and want to provide yourself with an adequate amount of omega-3, then 500 milligrams daily should suffice.

When buying fish oil supplements, check the label, because the dosage is based on the amount of EPA and DHA each capsule contains and not the actual amount of fish oil. Most fish oil supplements contain 180 milligrams of EPA and 120 of DHA in each capsule.

If you do not want to take fish oil but still desire an omega-3 supplement, there are some manufacturers who make a DHA or EPA vegetarian omega-3 supplement from algae or seaweed. The capsules themselves are also from a nonanimal source, so they are a viable alternative for vegetarians and vegans.

If you have diabetes, you are likely unable to convert ALA into EPA and DHA, so an omega-3 supplement composed of flaxseed oil will not help you get the omega-3s you need. Also, some people with type 2 diabetes experience a dramatic rise in their blood sugar levels when they take fish oil supplements, so be sure to talk to your health-care adviser before taking omega-3 supplements. Likewise, do not begin taking omega-3 supplements if you are also taking blood thinners (e.g., aspirin, clopedigrel, warfarin), because the fatty acid acts as a blood thinner, too.

Side effects of omega-3 supplements are not common, although some people experience mild diarrhea or stomach upset when they first start taking the capsules.

PTEROSTILBENE

If you've never heard of pterostilbene (the *p* is silent: tero *still*-bean) before now, you are not alone, but word is spreading. That's because this derivative of resveratrol (which is also discussed in this chapter) shows promise in enhancing life span and has been shown to protect against age-related diseases such as Alzheimer's disease.

Pterostilbene is a type of polyphenol called a stilbenoid, a substance synthesized by plants in response to infectious attacks. This characteristic makes pterostilbene and other stilbenoids (such as resveratrol) excellent nutrients to support the immune system, among other benefits. Blueberries and grapes contain small amounts of pterostilbene, but the most abundant and cost-effective source is from the heartwood and bark of the Indian kino tree (*Pterocarpus marsupium*), which grows in India and Sri Lanka.

Pterostilbene, Health, and Aging

Although pterostilbene and resveratrol have nearly identical structures, the small differences between the two substances mean they are capable of providing different benefits. Pterostilbene's structure makes it easier for your body to absorb it and lets it stay in your body for an extended time, which in turn provides you with more advantages. Here are a few of them:

- In a head-to-head animal study of pterostilbene and resveratrol, pterostilbene, but not resveratrol, had a positive impact on stress, inflammation, and Alzheimer's disease. Researchers also report that working memory is correlated with pterostilbene levels in the hippocampus, the area of the brain involved with the formation, organization, and storage of memory.

- Animal research on *Pterocarpus marsupium* indicates that pterostilbene can lower total cholesterol and "bad" (lipoprotein low-density, LDL) cholesterol levels, rejuvenate beta cells in the pancreas (which can help people with type 2 diabetes), and reduce blood sugar and inflammation in type 2 diabetes, all benefits that can promote longevity. In fact, studies showed that pterostilbene could lower LDL cholesterol and triglycerides (a type of fat associated with cardiovascular disease) in a way similar to a drug called ciprofibrate. However, since ciprofibrate has side effects such as nausea and muscle pain and pterostilbene does not, the natural supplement seems to be a better choice.

- In Step 1, I discuss a toxin called AGEs—advanced glycation end products—substances associated with high blood sugar and diabetes that speed up the decline of the kidneys, heart, and eyes. The good news about pterostilbene is that it can directly block the formation of AGEs and it has also prevented damage to the liver and kidneys in diabetic rats.

- Worried about age-related atherosclerosis? Pterostilbene "may be a potential anti-proliferative agent for the treatment of atherosclerosis," according to a recent study by Park et al. in *Vascular Pharmacology*. And when it comes to fighting cancer, pterostilbene has shown some impressive study results. In fact, because pterostilbene is such a small molecule it can easily enter cancer cells, where it appears to destroy the cell's membrane and DNA and cause the cell to self-destruct. These findings have been shown in studies of breast, prostate, pancreatic, colon, lung, liver, and skin cancers.

- Pterostilbene also seems to have an affinity for the digestive tract, and a number of studies, including one from the National Kaohsiung Marine University in Taiwan, reported "their findings strongly suggested the chemopreventive potential of dietary administration of pterostilbene against colonic tumorigenesis [formation of tumors in the colon]." The study's authors, Chiou et al. went so far as to say that "pterostilbene was a more potent chemopreventive agent than resveratrol for the prevention of colon cancer." Although resveratrol has plenty of age-defying benefits of its own, pterostilbene appears, at least for now, to possess an ability to specifically target colon cancer, a disease that kills more than fifty thousand Americans every year.

- Yet another age-defying advantage of pterostilbene is its ability to mimic the benefits of calorie restriction (which is discussed in Step 1) on a molecular level. Studies indicate that pterostilbene can directly modulate the same genes impacted by calorie restriction—genes that protect the body against various age-related degenerative diseases, cancer-causing genes, and up-regulating genes that restrict cancer development. Pterostilbene can also suppress genes involved with inflammation-related conditions such as atherosclerosis and chronic inflammatory diseases and up-regulate brain proteins involved in memory.

How to Take Pterostilbene

Because pterostilbene and resveratrol are closely related and work synergistically, it is common to see both of these nutrients in the same supplement. You can, however, get pterostilbene-only supplements. Although no recommended intake has been established, a typical dose is 25 to 100 milligrams daily. Thus far no significant side effects have been reported among people using pterostilbene.

RESVERATROL

Resveratrol, a cousin of pterostilbene and an antioxidant that is found in red grapes and most berries, piqued the interest of scientists in the early 1990s when it was first reported in red wine. Almost immediately, there was speculation that the antioxidant resveratrol could explain the French Paradox—the observation that death from coronary heart disease remains low in the French even though many of them smoke and their diet is high in saturated fat. The French also tend to drink a lot of red wine, and this beverage contains resveratrol and high levels of flavonoids, all of which have potent antioxidant activity.

Subsequent studies have largely supported health benefit claims for resveratrol, but the field has now grown to include its possible and potential impact on cancer and aging, along with heart disease.

Resveratrol, Health, and Aging

If you believe some of the claims made by producers of resveratrol supplements, you'd think the phytonutrient is a fountain of youth. Although such a lofty label does not belong on resveratrol, the antioxidant can provide some anti-aging benefits, and they're supported by scientific studies. Thus far, most of the research has involved animals rather than people, but the findings have implications for people.

- Promising results have come out of studies of resveratrol in the fight against breast cancer, as well as prostate, pancreatic, and thyroid cancers.

- Resveratrol may help prevent blood clots as well as damage to your blood vessels, properties that are critical in the prevention of cardiovascular diseases.

- Animal study results suggest resveratrol may protect individuals from diabetes and obesity.

- Resveratrol may also reduce levels of "bad" (LDL) cholesterol.

- Regarding longevity, resveratrol studies have shown the antioxidant can extend the lives of some species, including worms, fish, and fruit flies. But can it do the same for people? This question has yet to be answered. However, an aging study done in mice discovered that a low dose of resveratrol modified gene expression in the brain, heart, and skeletal muscle in ways similar to that caused by calorie restriction (see Step 1), which has been shown to extend life span in humans. The resveratrol also suppressed the age-related decline in heart function in the study. In a University of Connecticut School of Medicine review of resveratrol and the heart, the investigators reported "it appears that resveratrol can induce the expression of several longevity genes including Sirt1, Sirt3, Sirt4, Fox01, Foxo3a and PBEF and prevent aging-related decline in cardiovascular functioning including cholesterol level and inflammatory response," even though thus far it has not been shown to affect the life span of mice. Generally, findings like these provide hope and evidence that resveratrol may be helpful in fighting the effects of aging in people.

How to Take Resveratrol Supplements

Even though red wine contains resveratrol, you would need to drink a large amount per day to appreciate the level of the phytonutrient to protect your cardiovascular health and other benefits. According to Xi Zhao-Wilson, PhD, one fluid ounce of red wine contains an average of 90 micrograms of resveratrol, so the typical 5-ounce serving would give you about 450 micrograms. A suggested intake of resveratrol is 20 milligrams (or 20,000 micrograms), so clearly the safer and more sober choice is a supplement!

In some studies, mice showed favorable antiaging changes in gene expression when they were given the human equivalent of 20 milligrams of resveratrol per day. Yet many resveratrol supplements on the market contain much higher amounts of the phytonutrient, usually 500 milligrams. At this point, there is no clear decision on the best dose of resveratrol, although the good news is, there are no known adverse effects associated with taking the supplement. A small study in ten people found that a single dose up to 5 grams did not cause any serious effects.

A resveratrol supplement may be taken alone or in combination with its close cousin pterostilbene. (See "Pterostilbene" in this chapter.) Most of the resveratrol supplements sold in the United States are made of extracts of the root of *Polygonum cuspidatum,* which is also known as Hu Zhang. You can also purchase red wine extracts and red grape extracts that contain resveratrol and other polyphenols.

VITAMIN D

Vitamin D is a fat-soluble vitamin that is found naturally in only a few foods, although it is added to some such as milk and cereals. The main source of vitamin D is ultraviolet rays from sunlight, which trigger the production of vitamin D when they strike the skin.

So you get enough of the sunshine vitamin? Many people don't, especially as they get older and worry (rightfully so) about sun exposure and the risk of skin cancer. You can reach a healthy balance between sun exposure and skin cancer risk: the general recommendation for making enough vitamin D is ten to fifteen minutes per day of sun exposure during peak hours (10 AM to 2 PM) at least four days per week. If, however, you don't have much exposure to the sun because of lifestyle or geographic location, then a vitamin D supplement may be appropriate.

Vitamin D, Health, and Aging

Vitamin D is a necessary nutrient for many reasons, including the fact that it helps your body absorb calcium. Without sufficient vitamin D, your body would excrete as waste much of the calcium you take in, so vitamin D is critical for bone health and for prevention of osteoporosis. But the benefits of this vitamin don't stop there.

- Vitamin D is a potent antioxidant that fights free radicals involved in aging.

- Ongoing research indicates that vitamin D is likely a neuroactive steroid that plays a significant role in adult brain function. A study from the University of Queensland, Australia, notes that deficiencies of vitamin D have been associated with cognitive decline, depression, Alzheimer's disease, and Parkinson's disease. Other research involving more than thirty-three hundred older adults found that a deficiency of vitamin D was associated with an increased risk of cognitive impairment.

- Studies suggest vitamin D can reduce inflammation associated with arthritis and other inflammatory conditions, including heart disease.

- When looking at cardiovascular disease, research indicates that vitamin D deficiency is associated with a significant risk of cardiovascular disease and poorer survival. A large (more than ten thousand patients) University of Kansas Medical Center and Hospital study reported that supplementation with vitamin D was associated with better survival. A Harvard Medical School study followed 1,739 people (mean age 59 years) for up to 7.6 years and concluded that those who were deficient in vitamin D_3 had twice the risk of a heart attack, stroke, or heart failure as healthy participants.

- If you want your immune system to function at its best, make sure you get sufficient vitamin D. Studies indicate that arming your immune system with vitamin D can help protect against disorders like the common cold and flu.

- If you struggle with asthma, and many adults do, then maintaining an adequate vitamin D level could be beneficial, as the vitamin may reduce the severity and frequency of asthma symptoms.

- Vitamin D appears to be beneficial in preventing rheumatoid arthritis in women. For men the jury is still out, but chances are maintaining a healthy level of vitamin D certainly won't hurt!

- Adequate levels of vitamin D have been shown to

significantly lower your risk of developing cancer, when compared with people who have lower levels.

How to Take Vitamin D Supplements

If sunshine and foods are not your main sources of vitamin D, then a supplement is in order. While the consensus among experts is that vitamin D is critical, they don't always agree on the best form to take or how much. When shopping for vitamin D, you'll likely see two types—D_2 and D_3. Most scientists say these two types are equally effective in the bloodstream, although some insist D_3 is about three times more potent than the former and so is the preferred form.

Vitamin D deficiency is considered to be common; therefore, some experts urge people to take amounts greater than the 600 International Units (IUs) recommended for adults up to age 70 and the 800 IUs for those older than 70. The National Osteoporosis Foundation recommends 800 to 1,000 IUs of vitamin D_3 for adults older than 50.

A good rule of thumb is to first have a blood test to determine your vitamin D level. Generally, clinicians in the United States believe that a vitamin D level at or greater than 20 nanograms per milliliter (ng/mL) is adequate for health. (The Vitamin D Council, however, advocates levels of 50 to 80 ng/mL, which will require you to take more than 800 to 1,000 IUs daily.) Your doctor can order a vitamin D test for you, or you can order your own test online—no doctor necessary. In either case, discuss the results of your test with your physician to determine if you need to take a supplement and, if so, the best dose for your needs.

STEP 7

Connect with Your World

According to a massive research review of 148 studies conducted by two universities, a healthy social life could be as beneficial to your long-term health and longevity as not smoking. In fact, the researchers found that people who had poor social connections had on average 50 percent higher chances of dying during the study's follow-up period (7.5 years) than did people who had active social lives. The message is clear: Socialize! Mingle! Connect with people and your world!

Some people are naturally more outgoing and social than others, and if you are one of those individuals then you probably find it easy to reach out to people you don't know, whether you have just moved to a new city or started a new job or are in a social setting where you don't know anyone.

Or you may be someone who finds it difficult to walk into a situation where you don't know anyone or to start a conversation with a stranger. For some people, these social skills decline over the years if they lose friends, family members, and their partner—people whom they may have counted on to help make social connections easier for them.

Whether initiating and maintaining social connections is easy or challenging for you, they are a critical part of an age-defying program. In this chapter you will discover the benefits of reaching out and connecting with your world—with people, animals, and nature—and lots of suggestions on how to make those connections. Included are tips ranging from how to broaden your social circle to the importance of touch and sexual intimacy.

HOW SOCIAL CONNECTIONS BENEFIT HEALTH AND DEFY AGING

How "social" are you? Do you talk, mingle, or interact with several people every day? Do you seek out new acquaintances and social opportunities? The typical way to measure social interaction is to identify how often people talk on the phone with other people, how often they get together with them, and how many people they share their feelings with.

When you socialize with people, you may be protecting your brain at the same time, because socializing is a type of mental exercise that stimulates your brain and forces it to respond. People can be challenging to deal with, be it their personalities, the topics discussed, or other factors, and so socializing prods your brain into action.

This idea is supported by much evidence. For example, a U.S. team found that talking to another person for as little as ten minutes a day can improve your memory. The higher your level of social interaction, the better your cognitive functioning will be, according to Harvard researchers. They discovered that people who had at least five social ties, such as a church group or other organized social gathering, or who visited people regularly, volunteered, or talked on the phone with family or friends were less likely to experience a decline in cognitive functioning than people who had no social interactions.

In another study, researchers who evaluated 2,575 adults older than 65 showed that those who had few social contacts over a three-year period were more likely to die than those who had a fuller social life. When individuals increased the number of social contacts from a few to many more, they also enjoyed an improvement in longevity that rivaled that of their peers who already had a great number of social relationships.

The social fabric is a warm and comforting one. Your personal relationships with others, whether they are family, dear friends, acquaintances, coworkers, or neighbors, can provide you with a sense of love, security, belonging, and gratitude. These positive feelings have a significant beneficial impact on both physical and mental/emotional health and thus help support and promote your efforts to stay younger, healthier, and smarter longer.

A Big Study on Loneliness

I am returning for a moment to the large study with which I opened this chapter, because the findings are an excellent representation of the importance of social relationships and friendships on mortality. The meta-analysis conducted by experts at Brigham Young University included data from more than three hundred thousand people who participated in nearly 150 studies. They were asked questions such as "Do you feel lonely?" "Do you have people you can count on in times of need?" and "Do you live alone?"

An evaluation of the answers revealed that people who had adequate or high social relationships with family, friends, coworkers and colleagues, or neighbors were 50 percent more likely to survive than their friendless peers. The researchers even likened being socially isolated or having low social interactions with being as harmful as:

- Never exercising

- Smoking fifteen cigarettes per day

- Being an alcoholic

- Being obese—in fact, being a loner is twice as dangerous as being excessively overweight

It is generally easier to maintain a high level of social contact when you are in the workforce, attend school, have a family to go home to every night, keep in regular contact with old friends, and are active in a social group such as a church, PTA, or political organization. But relationships are organic, and so they are in a state of constant flux and change, which in turn alters the integrity and makeup of your social fabric. Changes come in many forms: you or your friends or family move, your children leave home, illness may strike you or loved ones, divorce and other personal dynamics may permanently change your relationships with others, you retire and lose your coworker connections, people you care about die—these are the realities that can alter and reduce your connections with other people.

Given that maintaining social relationships is so important, how many friends and acquaintances should you have to help defy aging? According to Julianne Holt-Lunstad, PhD, one of the study's coauthors, "There's been this notion that it's just those people who are 100% socially isolated who are at risk, and that if you have one friend, you are OK. But this isn't the case. People who have more, or more complex, social resources vs. people who have less, have higher rates of survival."

That means getting and staying socially active and connected is good for your longevity. So let's get started.

MAKING NEW CONTACTS

Helena is a 56-year-old claims adjuster who was recently divorced. Although she got half of nearly everything in the divorce settlement, one thing she didn't get half of was the friendships she and her ex-husband, Frank, had cultivated over the years. Most of their socializing had involved Frank's business associates and their spouses, and so now Helena was left out in the cold. Her one dear friend lived several hundred miles away, and Helena's two grown children lived across the country.

Except for a few coworkers, Helena felt isolated and lonely, and she began withdrawing into herself. The lonelier she felt, the more she sought solitude, and she became depressed.

Helena's situation is not unusual. A change or tear in people's social fabric can completely disrupt their lives and drive them to socialize less and less, until some nearly isolate themselves. This tendency increases as people get older and/or when additional tears occur, such as loss of social contacts through death, divorce, retirement, moving, or disagreements.

In Helena's case, she got some help from her best friend, Caroline, who heard the sadness and loneliness in her friend's voice and words over the phone. One day Caroline appeared on Helena's doorstep, greeting her friend with the words, "It's time to get you back into the world."

One critical part of maintaining a strong social fabric is being willing to take the first step to pull the threads together when something tears them apart. If you are fortunate enough to have a friend like Caroline in your life, he or she may provide the prompt you need to remain social in your world. (Likewise, if you know someone who is withdrawing socially, you might consider helping him or her reenter the world.) If you don't, then it's up to you to make sure you take the steps necessary to remain engaged in society.

Just like other journeys in life, the first step is usually the hardest one to take. To lessen your apprehension, take small steps at first and choose situations that are the most comfortable for you. If possible, find an acquaintance, neighbor, coworker, or family member to accompany you. If you have a trusted friend or family member with whom you can share your fears and insecurities about reaching out to make social connections, discuss them. Even if this individual does not live nearby and cannot accompany you, moral support and understanding can be great motivators.

Where to Make Social Connections

Here are some social situations where you can meet people or at least mingle, perhaps share common interests and goals, get in tune with what is happening in your neighborhood or community, and feel more a part of the greater social fabric of your world. Most of these opportunities are free; a few may have a minimal charge.

- **Lectures.** Many public libraries offer free lectures on a variety of topics. Check the calendar of events for your local libraries as well as flyers and announcements in their lobbies. Other venues for lectures may include community centers, natural food stores (a good source of nutritional talks), community colleges and universities, and businesses that are trying to sell a service or product. If you attend a lecture given by someone in the latter group, be prepared for some sales pressure!

- **Grand openings.** New stores or services in your community may hold a grand opening with demonstrations, samples, and information. They provide an opportunity to meet other people and learn more about your community.

- **Block parties.** Neighborhood block parties are a great place to meet your neighbors. If you are new to a community or if you just don't know many people, here is a great way to socialize.

- **Yard sales.** If a neighbor is having a yard sale, you can either (1) buy something (if you are really interested), (2) stop by when business is slow, introduce yourself, and chat, and/or (3) stop by, chat, and offer to help (i.e., be "neighborly"). Even if the yard sale is not in your neighborhood and you enjoy such sales, visiting some may give you an opportunity to talk about specific items with other people. Strike up a conversation about collecting old records, glassware, or dolls.

- **Flea markets.** Flea markets may present you with many chances to initiate conversations with vendors as well as other shoppers. Even though you likely won't establish any lasting friendships, you have a chance to keep up your social skills and meet a variety of people, if only briefly.

- **Farmers' markets.** An ideal place to meet your neighbors—both those who provide the produce and those who shop for it. Initiate conversations with questions about local produce, gardening tips, recipes, and related topics.

- **Fairs, parades, and festivals.** Local fairs, parades, and festivals allow you to better know businesses and people in your community. If you see someone you know—a neighbor or acquaintance— stop and talk for a few minutes rather than just waving or passing him or her by.

- **Dog parks.** You don't need to own a dog to go to a dog park, but if you have a pooch a dog park is a great place to meet people. "Dog people" love to talk about their pets, and if all goes well you and your new acquaintances may get beyond discussions of favorite dog biscuits and bathing techniques to more "human" topics.

- **Malls.** Yes, malls can be fairly anonymous, but they also can offer chances to chat with salespeople and shoppers or to participate in events held there, including demonstrations, information fairs, and entertainment events. Some large malls are venues for mall walkers: an organized group of people who use the safe and weatherproof security of an indoor mall to enjoy walking as a group, typically before the mall opens.

- **Book and poetry readings.** Big bookstores, small local bookstores, colleges, coffee shops, and libraries are common venues for book and poetry readings. These are good venues to share ideas with people who are interested in a given topic or author.

- **Demonstrations.** Cooking, do-it-yourself home repairs, decorating ideas, and more may be offered at malls, home supply stores, craft stores, and community centers. Again, you may meet people with similar interests.

Ways to Broaden Your Social Connections

I'm not done yet with suggestions on how to trigger or initiate social interactions. Some of these ideas can be incorporated into each opportunity you have—like those mentioned under "Where to Make Social Connections."

- **Volunteer.** Every community, town, and city has volunteer opportunities. From your local library to soup kitchens, animal shelters, hospitals, homeless shelters, literacy programs, museums, children's programs, and historical societies, there are scores of groups, organizations, and causes that would welcome your time and energy. And the age-defying benefits are significant: people who volunteer, and especially older adults, "may enjoy good health and longevity because being useful to others instills a sense of being needed and valued," according to researchers at the University of Guelph. Washington University experts have noted that "there is good evidence of a reciprocal relationship between volunteering and well-being."

- **Smile.** A smile is the universal language. Without speaking a word, a smile says "hello," "welcome," and "let's share—at least this moment." A smile is an icebreaker and suggests you are receptive to conversation. That's not to say the person to whom you have directed your smile will reciprocate, but if he or she does then you have opened a door—so walk on through!

- **Call up old friends and acquaintances.** If you look at your address book and say to yourself, "Gee, I haven't spoken with so-and-so for such a long time," why haven't you? These same people could be looking at their contact list and saying the same thing about you. Take the first step and stay in touch. They will likely appreciate it, and you could reestablish communication and a friendship. If the phone number you have is no longer in service (lots of people have dropped landlines in favor of cell phones), then mail them a note or card saying you'd like to hear from them and give your contact information—phone, address, and e-mail.

- **Make eye contact.** It's surprising how many people don't look you in the eyes when they talk to you. Making eye contact is a way to show you are interested in what someone is saying and that you are listening. Try it next time you meet someone, and then keep on doing it!

- **Introduce yourself.** Did you read the long list of "Where to Make Social Connections"? Many of them are situations in which you will likely not know anyone, so you should introduce yourself. Take a deep breath, say "Hello, I'm so-and so," and start the conversation with something that elicits a response, based on the circumstances. For example: "I'm new to this area." Followed by: "Where are the best places to shop for _____?" or "Have you heard this speaker before?" or "Can you tell me about other bookstores in the area?"

- **Be a mentor.** Put your life skills to work by helping others as a mentor. Perhaps you have a business background, have worked with kids (your own count, too!), have artistic talents, have played or coached sports, have organized social or business events, or have any number of other skills. As a mentor, you can help build a child's self-esteem, help him or her with life and academic skills, and encourage positive behaviors. Mentoring opportunities may be available through schools and churches in your area, organizations like Big Brothers Big Sisters, or through a national mentoring organization called MENTOR (http://www .mentoring.org/).

- **Participate in group activities.** Find a group in your area that mirrors some of your interests. You may be drawn to a church or spiritual group, political party, or social cause. Perhaps you are interested in photography, writing, bird-watching, embroidery, poetry, animal welfare, music, bridge, antiques, painting . . . the list is endless. Attend a meeting or function and learn more about the group by talking with other group members and visiting their Web site. If the experience feels right, then you've made a match! If not, try another group.

- **Practice social networking.** If you are not already part of the social networking scene, it may be time to try it. MySpace, Facebook, Bebo, Friendster,

and others are among the most commonly used
sites. Chances are good you know someone who is
using at least one of these networking sites and he
or she can help you get started. Social networking
isn't just for individuals. Many organizations and
groups have a Facebook page, where you can keep
updated on activities and news, and you may connect with some new people and events through the
Web site. Then it's up to you to make the connection face-to-face!

Maintain "Old" Social Connections

Maintaining relationships with anyone is a matter of give-
and-take, and it requires some effort—and that's true
whether they are your life partner, your child, your best
friend, or a coworker and whether they are still physically in
your life or have moved away. Let's consider the former for
a moment.

It's easy to get caught up in the flurry of your life or to
become depressed and perhaps withdraw or take for granted
some of the people in your life. If that happens, both you
and the other people lose out on something very special.
The "effort" to keep your relationship healthy is a natural
extension of your caring and concern for each other. Perhaps
your lifestyle and schedule allow you to see your family and
friends daily or often, and that's great. If not, however, you
may need to set aside a specific time each day, every few
days, or once a week. Perhaps it's the walk you and your partner take each day, lunch with a coworker, or meeting for
coffee at a favorite café once a week with your best friend.

The day when a best friend, child, favorite neighbor, or
beloved family member moves far away can be a very dis-
tressing one, and the days, weeks, and months that follow
may never feel quite the same to you again. Your inability to
reach out and touch the person's hand, give him or her a hug,
go out together, or share a meal in your favorite restaurant
can be depressing.

But there are a number of ways to deal with the sense of loss and disconnection and, with modern technology, stay connected in new ways. And some of the old ways work well, too!

Here are some suggestions.

- **Use Skype.** This free Web-based videophone service allows you to see who you are talking to on your computer screen, but it also allows you to do much more, especially if you use a laptop or other portable device. For example:
  - Schedule a weekly coffee hour. Did you and your best friend always meet for coffee at a special café once a week? Then bring your laptop to the café, call your friend on Skype, and have that cup of coffee while he or she enjoys his or hers on the other end of the conversation.
  - Share a new location. If someone special has moved away, he or she can use Skype to show you around his or her new home or neighborhood. The laptop or device can be carried from room to room or any location to show you his or her new surroundings.
  - How does it look? If you would like your friend's or cousin's opinion on something you've bought—a dress, new piece of furniture, painting—connect with Skype and show him or her the item.
  - Join the party. Bring a computer or device to a family gathering, party, or other event and share the occasion with your loved one via Skype.

- **Play games online.** Did you know you can play games like chess, Scrabble, Monopoly, word games, puzzle games, and casino games online with someone anytime, anywhere in the world, while sitting at your computer? You can even have several different games going at the same time with different people. Web sites such as www.muchgames.com, www.spinchat.com, and www.pogo.com are just a few of the sites that offer these opportunities for you to stay in touch with people while having fun.

- **Use your cell phone for more than talking.** Calling your friends is great and highly recommended, but if you have a smartphone then you can do more, such as send text messages, photos, and e-mails.

- **Send a letter.** Yes, a real on-paper letter or card on which you have written a personal note or letter. Although high tech is okay, there's still something very warm and meaningful about getting a real letter you can hold in your hands or a card you can put on your nightstand.

- **Send e-mail cards.** Many Web sites offer free greeting cards for every occasion that you can personalize and send to your friends. Be prepared, however, to get caught up in looking at all the options. These e-cards are often animated, musical, and downright captivating and fun, so it may be hard to choose which one to send.

SOME OF MY BEST FRIENDS ARE ANIMALS

I know an older woman, Becky, who is divorced, lives alone, and doesn't have a wide circle of human friends. But she is not lacking for friendship, for as she says, "Some of my best friends are animals."

Becky shares her home with only two cats, Maxwell and Orwell, but her wider social network includes dozens of cats and dogs, as well as owls, hawks, and the occasional raccoon. You see, Becky is a volunteer at a no-kill animal shelter two afternoons a week and she also donates her time to a wild animal sanctuary on the weekends. Her love of animals tame and wild was her open door to a very active and fulfilling social network of human, furry, and feathered friends. "I enjoy my time with the animals, I feel like I'm accomplishing so much, and it's great spending time with people who share my interests."

Animals, Health, and Aging

More than a quarter century of scientific research supports the belief that establishing and maintaining relationships with animals, especially pets, is beneficial for your health and longevity. Animals can help improve your cardiovascular health, decrease loneliness and depression, and reduce stress. Dog ownership (or being a "pet parent") can offer a reduction in blood pressure that is equal to reducing salt in your diet or cutting down on alcohol. Petting a dog or cat, interacting with pet birds, and even watching fish in an aquarium have been proven to provide cardiovascular benefits.

Research has shown, for example, that

- People who have suffered a heart attack have benefited from increased survival if they are dog parents.

- Heart rates go down when people pet a dog or watch fish.

- Elderly people experience reduced muscle tension and an increase in skin temperature when they watch fish in an aquarium.

- Risk factors for cardiovascular disease, including cholesterol, triglycerides, and systolic blood pressure, are reduced when people pet animals.

- Levels of the "happy" hormones—dopamine and endorphins—rise and levels of the stress hormone cortisol decline after a quiet thirty-minute session with a dog.

- Dog parents typically get more exercise because they need to walk their pet, and this can improve their cardiovascular health.

- One study even found a greater reduction in cardiovascular stress response when people were in the presence of a dog than with a spouse or friend.

- A study of Australian cat owners found that people who had cats scored better on psychological health tests than did nonowners.

- Recently widowed women who had pets experienced significantly fewer symptoms of physical and emotional problems and used less medication than widows who did not have pets.

Being a Pet Parent

If you have a dog, you are probably already aware of the "magnet" factor: take your dog for a walk most places and you will likely attract attention and, often, conversation as well. Dogs can be automatic icebreakers. Dog people, as they are affectionately called, tend to flock together, and the rising popularity of dog parks is an illustration of that phenomenon.

If acquiring a dog (or cat) is something you would like to do and you are physically and financially able to manage it, sharing your life with a pet can be a wonderful social booster, as well as a physical, emotional, and spiritual one. You will need to weigh the pros and cons of your choice and consider many factors, ranging from size and age to all that's involved in the animal's care.

If you do decide to become a pet parent, remember that animal shelters, including those run by the Humane Society and the SPCA, are full of wonderful dogs and cats of many ages, sizes, and breeds that desperately need a loving home. Adoption fees vary, and often older adults can adopt for a very low cost or even free of charge.

NATURE, HEALTH, AND AGING

Can interacting with nature improve your social skills and your physical and mental health? Absolutely, say scientists. According to a study conducted by Ming (Frances) Kuo, a professor at the University of Illinois at Urbana-Champaign, where she directs the Landscape and Human Health Laboratory, when people are deprived of green space their health suffers significantly, including feeling lonelier and having inadequate social support. She also noted that people who have access to nature have better cognitive functioning and mental health, as well as higher levels of physical activity and improved immune system functioning.

A large Dutch study that evaluated the medical records of more than 345,000 people found that those who lived within a half mile of a wooded area or park were less likely to experience anxiety disorder and depression than people who lived in more urbanized areas. Being in the company of trees can even boost your memory. A University of Michigan team gave a group of people a thirty-five-minute task that involved repeating many random numbers back to a facilitator in reverse order. The group was then divided into two: one went for a walk in an arboretum and the other went down a busy city street. When both groups returned from their break, they were asked to repeat the memory test. The people who had walked among nature performed nearly 20 percent better than those who walked the city streets.

Experiencing nature on your own and sharing your experiences with another person are both age-defying events. Being in a natural environment has a calming effect, which can make you feel more self-assured and social. And when you combine social interaction and a natural setting you get twice the benefit!

But what if the closest thing you have to a park, wooded area, beach, or nature trail is a painting on your wall? Then it's time to bring nature to you via books, DVDs, and photographs. Researchers found that people who looked at pictures of natural scenes performed better on cognitive tests than people who looked at urban scenes or even geometric patterns. So watch nature shows on TV, pop in a nature DVD, and to make the experience even better invite a friend to share the experience!

INTIMACY, HEALTH, AND AGING

Dr. Dean Ornish, whom I introduced in Step 1, may be best known for his work with diet and nutrition, but his research into the connection between intimacy, love, and longevity is both powerful and critically important. In his landmark book, *Love & Survival: The Scientific Basis for the Healing Power of Intimacy,* he describes "the increasing scientific evidence from my own research and from the studies of others that cause me to believe that love and intimacy are among the most powerful factors in health and illness, even though these ideas are largely ignored by the medical profession."

In fact, this guru of diet states that when it comes to love and intimacy "I am not aware of any other factor in medicine—not diet, not smoking, not exercise, not stress, not genetics, not drugs, not surgery—that has a greater impact on our quality of life, incidence of illness, and premature death from all causes."

Wow. Those are words you don't expect to hear from a conventional doctor of medicine. But do they have any relevance to your life? Let's see.

What Is Intimacy?

First, what is intimacy? Perhaps you think immediately of sexual intimacy, and that is certainly an essential part of it. But there is also the intimacy when you share your innermost thoughts, fears, and other feelings with another person or persons. You have already read about how important it is to have friends and social interactions for your health and longevity, and that is still true. However, there is more.

According to James W. Pennebaker, PhD, author of *Opening Up: The Healing Power of Confiding in Others,* who has conducted much work in the area of human interactions, "If you have had a trauma that you have not talked about with anyone, the number of friends you have is unrelated to your health. Social support only protects your health if you use it wisely. That is, if you have suffered a major upheaval in your life, talk to your friends about it. Merely having friends is not enough."

The extra ingredient you need is intimacy. This form of intimacy involves opening up your heart and allowing someone else to touch you in an emotional way. Although it is not physical touch, it can have a tangible impact. Do you have people in your life with whom you can share this type of intimacy? If you do, it is important that you maintain those relationships, even if these individuals have moved away. They may include your spouse or partner, a family member, child, or best friend, or perhaps a therapist or spiritual teacher. If you lose one or more of these intimate connections, as typically occurs when someone loses his or her spouse or partner, having one or more people you can rely on to share your fears and intimate thoughts is important for your well-being.

Touch and Sexual Intimacy

People and other mammals need food, air, and water to exist, but they need touch to thrive. When infants are deprived of touch, they do not develop normally. The need for caring, gentle physical touch continues throughout your life. Although way too many people have experienced abusive touch in their lives, which can make them uncomfortable or even unable to tolerate positive physical contact, it is important to have some type of intimate touch in your life. In fact, touch "is the first language we learn," according to University of California, Berkeley, professor of psychology Dacher Keltner, author of *Born to Be Good: The Science of a Meaningful Life,* and it is "our richest means of emotional expression" throughout our lifetime.

Touch is a powerful healing force. It can:

- **Improve your self-esteem.** When someone touches you in a caring way—a pat on the arm, walking hand in hand, a hug—it communicates that you are an important, worthwhile person.

- **Create a closer relationship.** Touching creates a bond with the other person and provides a support system.

- **Release calming hormones.** Researchers at Brigham Young University and the University of Utah report that nonsexual, supportive touch such as a neck or back massage and hugs reduces stress hormone levels and blood pressure while also enhancing oxytocin, a hormone that has calming effects.

Sexual intimacy and sexual activity are good for longevity, and that goes for adults of any age. During a March 2008 interview on ABC's *Good Morning America,* Drs. Michael Roizen, an anesthesiologist and internal medicine specialist at the Cleveland Clinic, and Mehmet Oz, a heart surgeon at NewYork-Presbyterian Hospital, said men who have sex three times a week can reduce their risk of heart attack and stroke by 50 percent. Women benefit as well: those who enjoy sex tend to live longer than those who don't.

Not only might you live longer, but you'll feel better, too, according to the doctors. They report that great sex can make a woman's body feel two to eight years younger and men who have 150 or more orgasms per year can feel the same way. One reason may be that orgasm helps relieve general pain.

So how can you stay in touch more?

- **Hug often.** This suggestion can be applied to grandchildren, friends, relatives, spouses, and even neighbors and acquaintances if both of you are comfortable with this show of affection.

- **Massage.** A massage does not have to be sexual in nature. One of the more loving gestures you can do for your spouse, parents, or child is to give them a foot or neck massage. If, however, you have a sexual partner, a massage can be a more intimate show of affection.

- **Be open with your partner.** If you are in a long-term relationship in which the physical contact has diminished, a frank, loving discussion with your partner about your need for more physical touch may bring some spark into your relationship.

Naturally, all touch should be exchanged in a way that is respectful of the boundaries of both people involved. Once that is established, however, a sympathetic or loving touch from a friend, lover, or family member can send a powerful and soothing message.

I want to close this chapter with a few words from two individuals. One is James J. Lynch, PhD, author of *The Broken Heart* and a pioneer in the study of relationships, loneliness, and health. He noted that "loneliness is one of the leading causes of death in this country and certainly a major factor in heart disease. It's interesting how words like *loneliness* and *love* were made to disappear from science and medicine, and in their place came phrases like 'mental stress' and 'social support.' There is something about those words that's threatening—*love* is certainly a word that is taboo in science."

The other is Carol Naber, an intuitive healer who lives in California. In *Love & Survival,* she is quoted as telling Dr. Ornish, "Healing is a journey, and we can experience it through our relationships with others."

Don't let *love* or *intimacy* be taboo in your life. Embrace other people, animals, and nature, and share intimate moments whenever you can. If you do, your chances of healing yourself and living a longer, more complete, and healthier life increase.

STEP 8

Clean Up Your Act

Today's high-tech, fast-paced world offers you a wealth of products, benefits, and services that are supposed to make your life easier and more stress-free and sometimes even healthier. However, convenience doesn't always translate into something positive, so along with the so-called advantages there are frequently many not-so-healthy and often hidden hazards. Consider something as seemingly innocuous as a plastic bottle of spring water. You know staying well hydrated is important, so you may carry bottled water with you in the car, when you go to the store, to work, to the gym, on a hike. But your intended healthful move may have unintended negative consequences: some water bottles contain harmful bisphenol A (BPA), a chemical that can disrupt hormone levels, and it could be leaching into your water, triggering changes in your body that contribute to aging.

BPA is only one of scores of substances present in the environment and in everyday items that can be hazardous to your health and drain months and years from your life. But they don't have to. You can clean up your act and add healthier years to your life if you know what hazards to look for, how to avoid them, how to get rid of them once they make their way into your body or your environment, and, when applicable, how to find healthy alternatives. Obviously I can't discuss all the toxins that can promote aging, so this chapter addresses some of the more common ones.

TOXINS STEAL YEARS FROM YOUR LIFE

Toxins and pollutants are everywhere: in your air, water, soil, furniture, food, clothing, even the walls of your house. So how can you *possibly* avoid all of them? Well, you can't, but you *can* make minor changes to your life that allow you to protect yourself from these hazards.

Environmental toxins steal years from your life because they can accumulate in your body and promote the formation of free radicals, those nasty molecules that are produced in the body during normal metabolism or when you are exposed to environmental toxins such as cigarette smoke, food additives, or mercury. When too many free radicals accumulate in the body, they attack healthy cells and cause them to age prematurely. All your body's cells can be damaged by free radicals—fat cells, the cells that line the walls of your arteries, your immune system cells, and more. That's why free-radical damage (also known as oxidation) is associated with aging and degenerative diseases such as cancer, heart disease, cataracts, and diabetes. Environmental pollutants affect people more as they age, and because the number of toxins is ever increasing their ability to rob you of precious health and years is growing as well.

You can fight back, but before you pick your fight you need to know your enemies. I've presented them in alphabetical order, so no one element has been given more weight than another.

BPA

When you open up a can of tomatoes, soup, or vegetables, you may be getting more than you bargained for. That extra something in the can may be bisphenol A (BPA), an industrial chemical used to make some plastics and resins. Epoxy resins are used to coat the inside of metal food cans, and the chemical can leach into your food. BPA is also found in polycarbonate plastics, which are commonly used in food and beverage containers.

The National Toxicology Program at the Department of Health and Human Services has stated it has "some concern" about the possible impact of BPA on the behavior, brain, and prostate gland of fetuses, infants, and children. Research has shown high levels of BPA in women who have a common condition called polycystic ovarian syndrome (PCOS). There is also growing concern over the role of BPA in breast cancer and type 2 diabetes and the possibility that exposure to the chemical causes insulin resistance, which leads to type 2 diabetes and congestive heart failure.

Overall, BPA is both a toxin to avoid and one over which you do have a lot of control. Here's what you can do:

- **Reduce or eliminate the use of canned foods.** Most food cans are lined with BPA-containing resin, and foods with high acidity, such as tomato products or those containing citrus, are most likely to cause release of BPA. As an alternative, buy fresh or frozen foods whenever possible. Items such as pasta sauces and soups are available in glass and boxes, which are BPA-free.

- **Use BPA-free products.** Polycarbonate plastic is usually clear, hard, and lightweight, and it may have a No. 3 or 7 recycling symbol on the bottom. Avoid these items. Instead, look for plastics that are marked BPA-free or avoid plastic items.

- **Don't microwave your food in plastic containers.** When you microwave polycarbonate plastics, the materials can break down over time and leach BPA into your food. Microwave your food in ceramic or glass containers.

- **Use alternatives.** Instead of plastic containers and serving dishes, use glass, porcelain, or stainless steel for hot foods and liquids. Make sure these items are not lined with plastics.

- **Replace your plastic water bottle.** Some water bottles are BPA-free, but to be environmentally friendly as well as health conscious use a stainless-steel water bottle (without a plastic lining).

Excitotoxins and Other Food Additives

The Standard American Diet (SAD) is composed of foods that are a minefield of food additives. From diet sodas to microwavable dinners, boxed macaroni and cheese, canned soups, salad dressings, breakfast cereals, and more, most people are consuming a host of food additives every day. Food producers routinely add substances such as artificial colorings, flavorings, and preservatives to foods to improve texture, color, flavor, and shelf life.

Unfortunately, most of these additives (added nutrients are usually an exception) do nothing to enhance or "add" to your health. On the contrary, they can have damaging effects on your body and mind, and promote aging. Here I look at food additives in general, but first, as a subgroup, a group known as excitotoxins is worthy of particular attention because they are especially common.

What Are Excitotoxins?
Did you enjoy a diet soda today? Chances are it contained the artificial sweetener aspartame. Have you had a bowl of canned soup recently? It likely contained hydrolyzed vegetable protein. Both of these substances, as well as monosodium glutamate (MSG) and a host of other compounds, are examples of excitotoxins, substances added to foods and beverages that stimulate your nerve cells, promote the aging process, and damage the brain.

Most excitotoxins are amino acids that interact with certain receptors in the brain in such a way they end up harming some brain cells. One of the most commonly recognized excitotoxins is glutamate, and MSG is the sodium salt of glutamate, which is the neurotransmitter most used by the brain. At very low concentrations, glutamate is good for your brain. But when concentrations get too high—more than 8 to 12 micrograms—neurons behave abnormally and begin to die. Excitotoxins also trigger the production of lots of free radicals, which promote aging.

If you eat processed foods, you are consuming excitotoxins, which are added to help improve flavor and appeal. However, you won't see them listed as such on the ingredient labels. Excitotoxins are disguised under names like natural flavoring, spices, textured protein, soy protein extract, MSG, and yeast extract, to name a few. (See "Excitotoxins.") They can be found in everything from soups to diet soft drinks, salad dressings, gravies, and frozen dinners. Excitotoxins in liquids are more readily absorbed by the body than those in solid foods.

Although your brain is designed to prevent harm from glutamate—a system called the blood-brain barrier—this protective barrier is not as effective if you consume too many excitotoxins. If you are a big fan of diet beverages and processed foods, you may be getting an excessive amount of excitotoxins. A few other factors also affect how well the excitotoxins can get past the blood-brain barrier. One of them is age: as you get older, your barrier becomes more porous and lets more of the foreign substances into your brain. Another factor is health issues: high blood pressure, diabetes, stroke, vitamin and mineral deficiencies, and certain infections can all compromise the blood-brain barrier.

Protect Yourself Against Excitotoxins
Consider the following tips to help protect yourself against excitotoxins:

- **Pass up processed foods.** Focus instead on whole, natural foods.

- **Know your poisons.** Become familiar with excito-toxins (see the list starting on this page), read food labels, and identify which foods to avoid.

- **Get enough magnesium.** This mineral can help prevent glutamates from overburdening receptors in the brain. People who have low magnesium levels are more likely to experience a negative reaction to excitotoxins, such as headache or severe digestive problems. Rich food sources of magnesium include green leafy vegetables, as well as whole grains, nuts, and beans.

- **Try omega-3 fatty acids.** These essential fats can block excitotoxins. The best sources of omega-3 fatty acids are cold-water fatty fish such as salmon, tuna, and herring (but read "Mercury") or fish oil supplements, which should come from a reputable company that provides mercury-free products.

- **Zero in on zinc.** This mineral plays a role in preventing excessive absorption of excitotoxins. If you are zinc deficient, you are allowing excitotoxins to get the better of you. Adults need 8 milligrams (females) to 11 milligrams (males) per day. The best whole, natural food sources of zinc include nuts and beans, while many cereals are fortified with zinc.

EXCITOTOXINS

Artificial sweeteners	Aspartic acid
Aspartame	Barley malt

Bouillon	Monopotassium glutamate
Carrageenan	MSG
Citric acid	Natural flavorings
Corn syrup	Pectin
Cysteine	Phosphoric acid
Disodium guanylate	Protein isolates and extracts
Disodium inosinate	Sodium citrate
Dry milk powders	Soy (anything that includes the word "soy")
Gelatin	
Glutamate	Textured protein
Glutamic acid	Vegetable gum and protein
Hydrolyzed ingredients	Whey protein
Malt extract and flavoring	Yeast (anything that includes the word "yeast")
Maltodextrin	

Food Additives Can Promote Aging

Although the negative impact of any one food additive may not be notable on its own, the more significant danger is the effect from consuming many of them over time. Artificial substances force the body to work harder to fight them, and food additives can speed up the aging process as well as contribute to chronic conditions associated with aging, such as diabetes, cancer, heart disease, and stroke.

Dozens of food additives may be harmful, even some of those rated GRAS—Generally Recognized As Safe—by the Food and Drug Administration (FDA). The following common additives are among those that should be avoided if possible if you'd like to add some healthy years to your life. Check product labels before you purchase foods, beverages, and even nutritional supplements!

- **Artificial and natural flavorings.** These additives may be better called mystery flavorings, because the food industry uses hundreds of different proprietary ingredients to mimic natural flavors. The only indication you may see on a label is "artificial flavoring" or "natural flavoring," but the real identify of the substance is a secret. What you don't know could harm you.

- **Artificial colorings.** According to the Center for Science in the Public Interest (CSPI), a nonprofit consumer advocacy group that champions for health and nutritional issues, all artificial colorings (blue 1 and 2, green 3, citrus red 2, red 3, red 40, yellow 5 and 6) should be avoided, even though the FDA has rated them as acceptable. The Center points out that animal studies indicate a risk of cancer associated with all artificial colorings and that they also pose a risk of allergic reactions for sensitive individuals.

- **Artificial sweeteners.** On the surface, using artificial sweeteners and choosing foods that contain them seems like a good idea if you are trying to lose weight or if you have diabetes. However, these additives (e.g., acesulfame-K, aspartame, saccharin) increase cravings for real sugar and can trigger overeating. Artificial sweeteners have also been linked to cancer and other health problems. Ace-sulfame-K, for example, causes DNA damage (which can lead to cancer) and affects the thyroid in animals. Aspartame (Equal, NutraSweet) has been linked to leukemia, lymphoma, and breast cancer in animals. The CSPI has noted that lifelong consumption of aspartame likely increases a person's risk of developing cancer and that everyone should avoid beverages and foods that contain it. In 1977, the FDA proposed that saccharin (Sweet 'n Low) be banned because it caused cancer in animals. Congress stepped in, however, and said it could be used if the foods had a warning label. In 2000, Congress passed a law allowing food manufacturers to remove the warning notice. Some experts still believe saccharin poses a cancer risk and recommend avoiding it.

- **Butylated hydroxyanisole (BHA).** Manufacturers add this ingredient to retard rancidity in fats, oils, and foods that contain oil. The U.S. Department of Health and Human Services considers BHA to be reasonably anticipated to be a human carcinogen, based on the results of animal studies, but the FDA does not agree and has announced that BHA is safe. Better safe than sorry.

- **Butylated hydroxytoluene (BHT).** Similar to BHA, BHT is used to retard rancidity in oils, and it is often found in cereals, potato chips, and chewing gum as well. Depending on the study, BHT has been found to increase or decrease the risk of cancer in animals. However, research has found residues of BHT in human fat, so it appears to accumulate in the body, which is probably not a good sign.

- **High fructose corn syrup (HFCS).** Use of high fructose corn syrup in processed and prepared foods is widespread because it is cheaper than sugar and has a very long shelf life. Although it is advertised as "natural," HFCS starts out as cornstarch and is then made sweeter using a process that converts the starch into glucose subunits, which are then transformed into fructose. HFCS is associated with an increased prevalence of obesity, insulin resistance, kidney diseases, high blood pressure, and heart disease, and it also can interfere with the function of a hormone called leptin, which regulates feelings of satiety. When leptin malfunctions, people keep eating even when they are full. HFCS is an additive to avoid.

- **Hydrogenated vegetable oil.** This is another name for trans fat, a synthetic fat associated with an increased risk of heart disease and stroke. Trans fat has been implicated as being even more hazardous than saturated fat when it comes to cutting your life short. The Harvard School of Public Health reported that trans fat has been causing about fifty thousand premature heart attack deaths per year. Look for hydrogenated vegetable oils in processed foods, including cereals. Nutrition Facts labels are required to list the amount of trans fat per serving, but this can be deceptive, since manufacturers can list a food as having 0 g trans fat if one serving contains less than 0.5 gram per serving. A food that claims "no trans fat" means the food is trans fat free.

- **Monosodium glutamate (MSG).** This flavor enhancer is added to thousands of processed foods, often under different names. Some of those names include yeast extract, hydrolyzed protein, caseinate, whey protein, and malt extract, among others.

- **Olestra.** This is a synthetic fat marketed as a no-fat additive. When you consume olestra, it passes through your digestive system without being absorbed and also reduces your body's ability to absorb nutrients from fruits and vegetables. Use of olestra can cause diarrhea, loose stools, flatulence, abdominal cramps, and other side effects.

- **Sodium nitrite and sodium nitrate.** These two chemicals are added to smoked meats such as bacon and sausage to preserve color and flavor. They can combine with chemicals in the digestive tract to form nitrosamine, a known carcinogen. Although food manufacturers now add ascorbic acid to processed meats to inhibit the formation of nitrosamine, some research still points to an increased risk of cancer associated with dietary nitrate and nitrite. A September 2011 study, for example, reported on a greater than 30 percent increased risk of ovarian cancer among women who got nitrites from animal food sources. Processed meats are already not recommended for other health reasons, and the presence of sodium nitrite and sodium nitrate is yet one more.

Mercury

Mercury is a heavy metal that can have a detrimental impact on the brain and the rest of the central nervous system. In the past, mercury thermometers were a significant concern because they could break and release the toxin, but mercury thermometers are rarely used today. The dangers of mercury are still a concern from several other sources, however, including silver-amalgam dental fillings (which are about 50 percent mercury), fish, and pollutants from coal-burning plants.

According to neurologist Dr. David Perlmutter, author of *The Better Brain Book,* "mercury does its dirty work by promoting free radical production and inflammation; this is the same process that causes normal brain degeneration, but mercury does it much faster." Therefore, exposure to mercury can accelerate the aging of your brain.

Once mercury gets into your body, it can be difficult to get rid of it. This toxin can gradually build up in your tissues and lead to a number of problems related to aging. Studies show that people with Alzheimer's disease, for example, often have up to three times more mercury in their bloodstream than people who don't have the disease. Chronic exposure to mercury has also been linked with mental disorders, autoimmune disorders, and lesions in the mouth.

Sources of Mercury

Mercury comes in three forms: inorganic salts, elemental mercury, and organic compounds (e.g., methylmercury), which is the most harmful form. While you absorb little to no inorganic or elemental mercury, your body can absorb 90 percent of the organic variety from the digestive tract. Fish protein is very efficient: it holds on to more than 90 percent of the methylmercury the fish consume (which often comes from industrial mercury dumped into rivers and streams and from eating smaller contaminated fish or vegetation), and even cooking does not eliminate it.

What about mercury from dental fillings? Fortunately, many dentists don't use amalgam fillings anymore and offer other options. However, because the mercury-containing fillings were the only available fillings for decades, most adults who have dental fillings have mercury in their mouths. The American Dental Association maintains that amalgams are safe, even though experts generally agree that mercury can leach into the mouth from the fillings from the force of chewing. What professionals don't agree on, however, is how much mercury escapes into the body and how dangerous it is.

How to Avoid Mercury

When it comes to amalgam fillings, you may choose to have them removed. However, amalgam extraction can be hazardous and expose you to great amounts of mercury if the fillings are not removed by a highly skilled professional. If you are considering amalgam removal, you should be extremely careful and extensively research the risks and benefits and get several professional opinions before proceeding.

If you eat fish and seafood, choose items that are most likely to contain the least amount of mercury or other toxins. A general rule is, the larger the fish, the longer it lives, and the more likely it eats other fish that are contaminated with mercury. Fish and seafood with a minimal amount of mercury and other toxins include anchovies, cod, herring, pollock, salmon, and sardines.

AIR POLLUTANTS

The jury is back on the association between polluted air and premature death and increased hospital admissions. Air pollutants can be a combination of many elements, including chemicals, metals, organic biological compounds, dust, and soil that emerge from smokestacks, forest fires, vehicles, unpaved roads, and the result of substances that combine and react in the atmosphere. Don't forget that the air in your home and office is likely populated with pollutants as well.

Air pollution damages the cardiovascular system, elevates homocysteine (an amino acid linked to an increased risk of heart disease), levels and increases both oxidative stress and inflammation throughout the body, which can lead to blood clots and various heart and circulation problems. The gathering evidence is making it clear that bad air is bad for your health.

Remember the earlier discussions in this book about telomeres? When you are exposed to air pollutants from vehicle exhaust, cell-damaging molecules called reactive oxygen species are formed and they speed up the shortening of telomeres. If you live or work in an area where you are exposed to traffic pollution, you are likely aging faster than you should. Fine particles, such as those found in diesel exhaust, are said to shorten the lives of seventy thousand Americans every year, while many more experience the negative effects of respiratory and cardiovascular disease triggered by the pollutants.

How to Avoid Air Pollution

Short of wearing a mask (which some people do and is recommended if air quality in your area reaches a bothersome level), there are several actions you can take to reduce your exposure to air pollutants, both outdoors and in your home and office. Some of these ideas arise from a study done at the University of Leeds, where experts evaluated air pollutants in a city setting.

- **Avoid parallel streets.** In an urban setting, this is especially important if you are walking, jogging, or biking. Air pollutants tend to accumulate in pockets created by closely positioned buildings. Therefore, avoid using parallel side streets rather than main streets, because side streets usually have less airflow, which permits air pollutants to gather.

- **Avoid or don't linger in intersections.** Long-idling vehicles make these locations a haven for air pollutants.

- **Choose clean-air mass transit when available.** Diesel-powered buses, trains, and ferries are common forms of transportation for commuters, but they are also significant sources of pollutants. An investigation by the Clean Air Task Force looked at exposure to diesel particles during typical commutes in four major American cities: Austin, Boston, New York City, and Columbus (Ohio). They found that diesel particle levels were four to eight times higher inside commuter cars, buses, and trains than in the outdoor air in the same cities. If you have an option, choose mass transit retrofitted with emission controls or, better yet, those that run on alternative fuels such as compressed natural gas or electric.

- **Protect your home against air pollutants.** The main pollutants in homes are gas and particle–releasing products (e.g., ovens, stoves, heating and cooling systems, air fresheners, asbestos, radon), which can be made worse by inadequate ventilation. While there can be short-term effects of these pollutants (e.g., dizziness, headache, irritation of the throat, skin, nose, and eyes), the long-term impact can rob you of years and include cancer, heart disease, and respiratory diseases. Some protective measures you can take include the following:
  - Change and/or clean the filters in your heating and cooling system regularly.
  - Have the ductwork cleaned at least once a year.
  - Use an air purifier/air cleaner.
  - Check for radon. This colorless and odorless gas can cause lung cancer. You can purchase a special device at a home supply store that can measure radon in your home.
  - Have gas appliances and systems checked for leaks.
  - Keep plants in your home that can help remove pollutants from the air. These include Boston ferns, Australian sword ferns, rubber plants, English ivy, and areca palm.
  - Avoid dry cleaning. The dry-cleaning industry uses toxic chemicals that linger on your clothing. If you do have clothes dry-cleaned, do not hang the clothes in your closet when you pick them up. Instead, remove the plastic and put the clothes outside for a day or two to allow the chemicals to dissipate.
  - Avoid use of conventional household cleaners, including ammonia and bleach, because they typically contain toxic chemicals. Alternatives

include baking soda, salt, and vinegar. For example, a "recipe" for an all-purpose household cleaner is one part water mixed with one part vinegar and placed in a spray bottle. Vinegar is a natural disinfectant, deodorizer, and cleaner while also safe to use on most surfaces, except marble. And no, your house won't smell like a salad, because the vinegar smell disappears when it dries. Need furniture polish? Mix 1 cup olive oil with $\frac{1}{2}$ cup lemon juice and you will have a nontoxic shine to your wood. There's no need to buy abrasive cleansers when pure baking soda will do the trick.

Cigarette Smoke

It's been established that cigarette smoking is a health hazard, so I don't need to tell you about the obvious link between smoking and lung cancer and that if you smoke you should stop immediately. Smoking is also a risk factor for many other diseases that can significantly shorten your life span, including heart disease, stroke, diabetes, and other forms of cancer.

But even if you don't smoke, you can still fall victim to secondhand smoke, also referred to as environmental tobacco smoke or passive smoke. In fact, in some ways secondhand smoke is more dangerous to your health than the smoke inhaled by a smoker, because as an innocent bystander you are exposed to sidestream smoke (smoke that comes from the end of a lighted cigarette) as well as mainstream smoke (smoke exhaled by the smoker). Sidestream smoke has higher concentrations of carcinogens than mainstream smoke, as well as smaller particles, which makes it easier for them to infiltrate your body's cells.

Exposure to secondhand smoke in nonsmokers has been linked to deaths from heart disease and lung cancer; reduced lung function; and chest discomfort, while the possibility that it increases the risk of breast cancer is still being investigated.

The only way to avoid secondhand smoke indoors is to ban all smoking in public buildings. Fortunately, antismoking laws are established in a growing number of cities and towns and some have even taken it one step further and banned smoking in some outdoor settings. Efforts to ventilate buildings or to separate smokers from nonsmokers are not totally effective. Avoidance of settings and situations where smoking is allowed thus remains the most effective way to protect yourself and your health.

ALCOHOL

Alcohol is one of those good-guy, bad-guy issues. First, let's look at the bad guy. With age, the body becomes more sensitive to the alcoholic effects of beer, wine, and spirits. Therefore, 2 glasses of merlot will likely have a greater impact on an older person than on someone who is younger, other factors being equal. If you have certain medical conditions, such as high blood pressure, diabetes, or ulcers, alcohol can make these health concerns worse.

Another consideration is your use of medications and supplements, some of which can cause dangerous reactions if you take them with alcohol. Since the chances of taking one or more medications increase with age, you also increase your risk of experiencing side effects if you choose to indulge. For example:

- Alcohol along with high doses of acetaminophen can increase your risk of liver damage.

- Your risk of bleeding in the stomach is greater if you take aspirin while drinking alcohol.

- Mixing alcohol with allergy and cold medications (e.g., antihistamines) can make you very sleepy, an extremely dangerous situation if you are driving.

- Some cough syrups and laxatives have high alcohol content and may increase your risk of side effects if you combine them with alcohol.

- Many prescription medications have drowsiness as a side effect, and adding alcohol to the picture will make that side effect worse.

Alcohol and Aging

One of the major concerns about drinking alcohol is how much it may impair judgment, coordination, and reaction time. If you are a heavy drinker, you are exposing yourself to an increased risk of developing some cancers, liver cirrhosis, immune system disorders, brain damage, problems with blood sugar levels, and adverse changes to your heart and blood vessels. It's not hard to figure out that none of these health challenges have a positive effect on prolonging your life.

Alcohol can have a few other nasty impacts on prolonging your life. Take calcium absorption, for example. Alcohol interferes with your ability to absorb calcium. Although a small amount of red wine contains antioxidants, including resveratrol (see Step 6), excessive amounts can leach the calcium from your body and bones and lead to low bone density and a greater risk of fractures.

If you're a woman, the effects of alcohol are worse than they are for a man. That's because women generally retain a higher blood alcohol level for a longer time, even when they drink the same amount as a man. Thus women are more likely to suffer from the harmful effects of alcohol.

Alcohol and the Brain

Your brain does not escape the effects of alcohol, either. Alcohol is a neurotoxin, which means it can damage parts of the brain. In the case of alcohol, the effect is usually on the frontal lobes of the brain, which can result in premature aging of the brain and Alzheimer-like symptoms, or a condition known as alcohol-related dementia.

Have you had a stressful day? Do you like to "de-stress" with a drink or two? Most people believe that an alcoholic drink can be a source of relaxation, but in reality, alcohol can increase stress hormone levels in the body and contribute to their negative effects on aging. Over time, prolonged exposure to stress hormones can cause your blood pressure to rise and suppress your immune system, two situations that are not conducive to longevity.

Alcohol and Your Skin

Alcohol can be cruel to your skin, because it can increase the rate at which your body excretes water, which results in dehydration, dry skin, and—you guessed it—wrinkles. Consuming alcohol limits the absorption of nutrients that help repair, maintain, and vitalize the skin, including vitamins A, C, E, B_1, B_2, B_3, and B_6 and omega-3 fatty acids. Alcohol also causes small blood vessels to expand, which can result in coarse skin and broken veins. The bottom line is that alcohol can age your skin more rapidly than not indulging, and the impact is worse for women than men.

Alcohol and Weight

One big complaint among aging adults is the tendency to put on extra pounds, which can contribute to health problems such as heart disease and stroke, as well as be a blow to self-esteem. Alcohol adds empty calories and fat around the abdomen. If you were to include just 1 beer or glass of wine per day to your current lifestyle, you would likely add fifteen pounds in one year unless you took steps to "work off" those extra calories. Are you prepared to also add a one-mile brisk walk to your daily schedule to offset 1 glass of wine? That's roughly what it will take to help prevent the creep of extra pounds around your middle.

Alcohol and Health Benefits

I'd be remiss if I didn't mention the health benefits associated with alcoholic beverages. If you are already a moderate drinker (defined as 1 drink daily for women and 2 for men), there's evidence this level of alcohol can enhance cardiovascular health, especially in middle age. However, moderate drinking may also increase your risk of colon and breast cancer. If you don't drink, the promise of possible benefits should not be viewed as a license to start. One the other end of the scale, if you are a heavy drinker, reducing your intake to a moderate level or stopping completely is recommended, as excessive alcohol consumption is associated with life-shortening conditions, such as heart disease, cirrhosis, cancer, and high blood pressure.

In the end, if you do drink, do so moderately and with knowledge of its potential aging effects. One drink equals 5 ounces of wine, 12 ounces of beer, and 1.5 ounces of hard liquor. You should also take a multivitamin supplement that contains 400 micrograms of folic acid, because alcohol can moderately deplete your body of folate (the natural form of folic acid).

DETOX YOUR BODY

Although your body naturally detoxifies itself, stress and the daily assault of pollutants prevent it from cleansing itself optimally. So even if you begin to avoid toxins right this very minute—which is encouraged!—a detox plan is an extra step you can take to help your body heal itself, allow your digestive system to relax, raise your energy level, and help prevent premature aging. While a detox plan does not cure any illness or disease, it can help your body function at a higher level so you can feel younger, healthier, and more energetic.

Choosing a Detox Plan

Specific detox plans vary, but generally they involve some fasting and a strict program of juices, water, fruits, and vegetables, as well as certain nutritional and herbal supplements. A detox plan usually lasts for seven to ten days, but you can do a shorter one. Before you begin any type of detox program, however, you should talk with a knowledgeable health-care professional, especially if you have any medical conditions (e.g., diabetes, anemia, kidney disease, heart disease) or are taking any medications that could be affected by such a plan.

Because your body eliminates toxins mainly through stool and urine, it's important for you to have regular bowel movements during a detox to prevent poisons released from your blood into your intestines from being reabsorbed into your body. Thus a detox plan that includes fiber from food or natural supplements (e.g., psyllium, triphala) is recommended. Without enough fluids, fiber cannot do its job, so be sure to drink lots of filtered water, herbal detox teas, or fresh vegetable juices as part of your plan.

Examples of detox plans include:

- **Water fast.** This is the most extreme type of detox plan, during which you drink water only. An all-water fast has several negatives, including the lack of any nutrition or fiber. If it is included as only a portion of a long detox plan, then a water fast may be acceptable.

- **Juice fast.** Both fresh fruit and vegetable juices (include the fiber!) and water are consumed during this fast.

- **Raw food diet.** You eat only raw foods or anything that has not been heated above 118 degrees Fahrenheit.

- **Commercial products.** There are a wide variety
  of packaged "plans" that include protein powders,
  nutrients, and herbal supplements. One of the more
  popular herbal remedies for detoxification is milk
  thistle, which contains a combination of substances
  known collectively as silymarin. Silymarin is a potent antioxidant that reduces free-radical production and can block toxins from binding to liver cell
  membrane receptors. Before using a milk thistle/
  silymarin detox program or any commercial plan,
  consult a knowledgeable health-care provider.

- **Master Cleanse diet.** This is a popular program
  that can be very difficult to follow, and it does not
  provide enough nutrients. The ten-day diet involves
  drinking a mixture of lemon juice, water, maple
  syrup, and cayenne pepper. An herbal laxative and
  a saltwater mixture are also included as part of the
  daily program.

A Sample Detox Plan

A simple, safe detoxification plan is one that provides small
amounts of clean, nutritious foods that allow your body to
rid itself of toxins gently and without disrupting your life.
Here is a sample detox plan that can be used for three or
more days (but talk to your doctor first). You will need a
high-speed food processor or juicer to make the smoothies.

The Fruity Detox

- Glass of warm spring water with juice of ½ lemon

- Breakfast: fruit and vegetable smoothie. There are
  many different combinations of fruits and vegetables you can use to make the smoothies. One example is given here. Combine all ingredients in your
  juicer or food processor:

- 1 cup spinach
- 1 cup strawberries
- 1 banana
- 2 cups water
- 1 tsp flaxseeds

- Snack (choose 1): an apple or pear, handful of raw almonds or walnuts, cucumber, celery, or carrot sticks

- Lunch: small salad with mixed greens, onions, carrots, cucumber, tomato; use fresh herbs and lemon juice as dressing.

- Afternoon snack: choose 1 from above or a smoothie.

- Dinner: Brown rice, barley, or quinoa with steamed beets; steamed greens (kale, mustard, turnip) with 1 tablespoon ground flaxseed, lemon juice, and olive oil; steamed zucchini or yellow squash with mushrooms tossed in olive oil and lemon juice.

Drink at least eight cups of purified water and/or green tea each day. Other tips to make your detox optimally effective include enjoying each meal and snack in a stress-free, unhurried manner, chewing your food thoroughly, and enhancing your experience with daily meditation.

STEP 9

Less Stress, More Life

"I'm under a lot of stress." "I feel stressed out!" "The stress is getting to me!" Most people are familiar with these sentiments . . . and perhaps you've felt or expressed these very feelings yourself. Stress is a part of life, and it can have both beneficial and detrimental effects on your health. Positive stress can be an invigorating and motivating force in your life. Buying a new house or a car you've always wanted can be both a stressful and joyful event, while breaking down on the highway and dealing with a broken refrigerator are negative situations.

For most people these represent mild to moderate stressful events. But when stress is chronic or persistent—when worries about your kids and your in-laws and your job and your mortgage and your marriage seem to go on and on without relief—stress takes on a life of its own. Then stress is a thief, robbing you of your physical and mental well-being and taking years off your life.

But it doesn't have to: if you learn how to anticipate and manage stress, you may slow the aging process and add years to your life. And that's what this chapter can help you do: discover how to handle stress in ways that fit into your lifestyle and add healthy years to your life.

STRESS PLUS ANXIETY = AGING!

Stress is a reaction to something that has happened. For example, you're driving to a meeting for which you're already ten minutes late and you suddenly find yourself in a traffic jam that's crawling at 5 miles an hour. Or you have to give a presentation in front of new clients and you're worried they may not like your proposal. Situations like these can be stressful, and your body automatically adapts and reacts to them. Your reaction is called the fight-or-flight or stress response, and it allows you to handle situations by heightening your senses and responses.

The situations I just presented are not dangerous ones, but your body is programmed to respond as if they were. If you're sitting in traffic you may strum your fingers on the steering wheel or feel the muscles in your neck and shoulders become tense. As you stand up at the podium to give your presentation you may sweat, your heart may beat fast, and your stomach may feel full of butterflies. In a short time, however, these reactions will pass and your body will return to its pre-stress level.

Stress is often accompanied by anxiety: while stress is a reaction to a *real* situation, anxiety is a general feeling of apprehension or fear that something *may* happen. Unfortunately, the body can't tell the difference between a real threat (stress) and the one the mind creates in a state of anxiety, and so the physical symptoms they can cause are similar. These symptoms can include:

- Rapid heartbeat

- Backache

- Nervous stomach

- Constipation or diarrhea

- Mood swings

- Problems falling asleep

- Sleeping too much or too little

- Excessive hair loss

- Sudden memory loss

- Muscle tension

- Excessive sweating

- Fatigue

- Excessive weight gain or loss

- Skin irritations

- Frequent urination

If you have other health problems, stress can make them worse. One common example is any type of gastrointestinal condition, such as gastritis, ulcers, or irritable bowel syndrome. Symptoms of these conditions are known to worsen in the presence of stress.

Stress Can Trigger Aging Habits

What are the healthiest ways to deal with stress? That's a topic I take up later in this chapter. Some people, however, choose ways that are not healthy or life sustaining. For example, a study released in November 2011 reported that some older adults (age 65 plus) are turning to smoking and alcohol, or increasing their use of same, in times of financial challenges. In fact, the researchers found that among older adults who said they were experiencing increasing financial strain older men were 30 percent more likely to take up heavy drinking than men who had remained financially stable. Women, on the other hand, were more likely to reduce their drinking when financially hard times hit.

Concerns about financial security, which are covered in Step 10, are understandably stressful, but adopting harmful activities to combat them is counterproductive and, in the end, more stressful and aging. Stress can also cause people to become depressed, which can lead to a loss of interest in physical activities, socializing, and eating right—all critical steps to living a longer, healthier life.

Chronic stress can damage your relationships with your partner, family, friends, and coworkers; it can make it difficult to concentrate and work; it can also jeopardize your immune system. Persistent or excessive stress can lead to aging rather than healthful habits, and that's a cycle you want to prevent or to break if it has already started.

STRESS SPEEDS UP THE AGING PROCESS

Scientists have physical evidence of the aging effects of stress on the body. The first study credited with directly linking stress with accelerated aging was published in 2004, and the subjects of the study were moms who were taking care of chronically ill children.

You can read the particulars of the study under "Stress, Telomeres, and Aging," on the next page but if you want the nutshell version, here it is: The researchers found physical evidence that chronic stress speeds up the shriveling of the ends of bundles of genes inside cells—the telomeres I've discussed in previous chapters—which shortens their life span and speeds up the body's aging process and deterioration. And from there, as the saying goes, it's all downhill—unless you learn to put the reins on those telomeres.

STRESS, TELOMERES, AND AGING

The landmark study linking chronic stress, aging, and telomeres involved thirty-nine women ages 20 to 50 who had been caring for a chronically ill child (e.g., with autism or cerebral palsy) for years. The comparison group consisted of nineteen women who had healthy children.

The researchers looked at the telomeres, which are the caps at the ends of chromosomes. Every time a cell divides, the telomeres get shorter, until eventually they get so short the cells can't divide anymore and they die. As more and more cells die, the process of aging becomes evident: muscles get weaker, the skin develops wrinkles, organ function slows down and fails, and brain function diminishes.

In this study, the longer a woman had been caring for a chronically ill child, the shorter her telomeres and the greater her levels of oxidative stress, a process in which molecules called free radicals damage the body's cells, including telomeres.

An important factor in this process is how much stress people perceive themselves to be under. The researchers found that women who perceived themselves to have the highest amount of stress had telomeres equivalent to someone ten years older when compared with women who perceived themselves to have the lowest levels of stress.[8]

Since the landmark study, much more research has been done regarding telomeres, stress, and aging. A more recent study (November 2011) appearing in *Biological Psychiatry* supported and added to previous findings, noting that higher levels of the stress hormone cortisol are associated with shorter telomeres in both healthy and depressed people but that people who are depressed tend to have shorter telomere lengths than their healthy counterparts.

Perception, Stress, Anxiety, and Aging

According to Thea Singer, author of *Stress Less: The New Science That Shows Women How to Rejuvenate the Body and the Mind,* you can reduce your stress level and reverse the signs of aging by changing your perception of and attitude toward stressful events. She noted in a *Chicago Tribune* interview that "it's the sense of being OUT of control that's our biggest stressor. If we think of it as something external, perceived stress, something we can't control, then we are a mess."

So the real harm associated with stress occurs if you become anxious in stressful situations. According to cell and molecular biologist Elizabeth Blackburn and health psychologist Elissa Epel, PhD, who pioneered research linking stress and immune cell aging, chronic stress accelerates the rate at which the body's cells age by a decade or more. Epel, along with Nobel Prize winner and cell and molecular biologist Elizabeth Blackburn, showed us that perceptions of stress, as well as actual stressful situations or thoughts, are associated with shorter telomeres. In other words, stress ages you at the cellular level.

The 3 A's of Stress Reduction

Even though you can't eliminate stress completely, you can reduce it to a comfortable or manageable level. You have more control over how you respond to stress than you may think. Avoiding stress is a matter of 3 A's: Adaptation, Attitude, and Actions.

Adaptation

- **Find or create better ways to manage your time.**
  Once you adapt your schedule to allow yourself
  time to complete the tasks you need to do along
  with those you want to do, you will experience less
  stress. You may need to keep a calendar and schedule your work, leisure, family, and personal time—
  sometimes seeing your life's activities on paper is
  an eye-opening experience and forces you to repri-
  oritize your life. If you begin to panic whenever
  you think about all the things you need to do, stop:
  write them down and prioritize them. In the process, you will reduce your stress and anxiety levels
  and feel more in control of your life.

- **Look for new ways to cope with stress.** That is a
  main focus of this chapter: suggesting ways you can
  manage and cope with stress in your life. Then take
  Action: try new stress-management techniques until you find ways that work for you.

Attitude

- **Work on changing how you think.** If you begin to
  worry about something, try to put the brakes on the
  anxiety. Work on letting go of things you can't
  change.

- **Look for the positive side of negative situations.**
  I'm not being Pollyanna—this attitude can really
  work. Negative thoughts can have a significant impact on your physical health, while positive ones
  can keep them at bay and bring down your stress
  level dramatically.

Action

- **Take care of yourself.** If you neglect your physical and mental health, your response to stress will deteriorate. Eat a nutritious diet, get sufficient sleep, don't smoke, limit your alcohol intake, and don't take any unnecessary medications.

- **Communicate your needs, concerns, and ideas with people you trust.** If you can establish a network of individuals to share your concerns with, you can manage stress better.

- **Practice stress-reducing or stress-management techniques regularly.** There are literally scores of things that you can do to manage and relieve stress, and I will present some effective options for you to consider.

ACTIONS: WAYS TO REDUCE STRESS

The stress in your life can come from a variety of sources and situations, and so it makes sense to make use of various stress-reducing tools not only to tackle the difficult times but also to help keep you balanced on a daily basis. Managing stress every day is important because aging waits for no one. That's why you need to try to stay one step ahead or at least in line with it! With that in mind, here are some suggestions for ways to reduce stress. Choose one or more to be part of your healthy lifestyle.

Meditation

The practice of meditation is thousands of years old, and while many people still practice this mind/body technique for spiritual purposes, it has also been widely accepted as a way to reduce and manage stress. One reason it has infiltrated

mainstream medicine is because it works, and there are scientific studies to support the claims.

Benefits of Meditation

Meditation offers lots of benefits for your mind, body, and
spirit:

- You can do it just about anywhere—you don't need
  to sit cross-legged on the floor in a quiet place. Once
  you learn how to meditate, you can practice while
  you're walking, waiting in line at the grocery store,
  eating lunch at work, and even in the middle of a
  stressful dinner with your in-laws.

- Meditation is simple and inexpensive and doesn't
  require any equipment.

- Just a few minutes a day can help bring down stress
  levels, but if you can spend fifteen minutes or more
  that's even better.

- You can increase your sense of self-awareness and
  gain new perspectives on situations that are bother-
  ing you.

- Meditation often sparks bouts of creativity.

- The feeling of calmness stays with you even after
  your meditation session is over.

- Meditation may help you better cope or even relieve
  symptoms associated with various medical conditions, such as allergies, anxiety disorders, asthma,
  depression, fatigue, heart disease, high blood pressure, pain, and sleep problems.

Does meditation have a physical impact on the body? According to a University of California, San Francisco (UCSF)

study, it may. Once again I am referring to telomeres. Scientists have shown that telomere length is linked to chronic stress and depression. Mindfulness meditation reduces stress arousal and may also increase positive-arousal states of being. The UCSF researchers have proposed that some types of meditation may promote telomere maintenance by reducing stress and stress arousal and increasing positive states of mind and hormonal factors associated with telomere well-being.

If you're being treated for a medical condition, meditation does not replace traditional care. However, it can be a useful complement to other therapies. If you do choose to meditate, tell your health-care provider, because you may be able to reduce or change medications or other treatments you are receiving.

Meditation can take many forms, including guided meditation and guided imagery, mindfulness, mantra, and walking meditation, which is a form of mindfulness. Since mindfulness meditation is one of the most common types and easy to learn, I explain it here, along with walking meditation.

Mindfulness Meditation

Mindfulness meditation (*samatha* meditation) is a practice in which you try to achieve a calm, stable mind. Tranquility is the natural state of the mind, and when you practice mindfulness meditation you can develop and strengthen that state of calmness until you can remain content much of the time. Of course, this takes practice, but as little as ten to twenty minutes a day over time can add many peaceful years to your life.

It's best to choose a quiet place to meditate, especially if you are new to the practice. Posture is also important: keeping your body erect, whether you are sitting or standing (as in walking meditation) facilitates the flow of energy through your body and your mind, allowing clearer thought processes.

With these thoughts in mind, here is a brief guide to mindfulness meditation:

- Choose a quiet spot where you can sit comfortably, either in a chair with your feet touching the ground or on a cushion on the floor with your legs crossed and your hands resting palms down on your thighs. Maintain an upright posture throughout the session.

- Keep your eyes open and gazing at a point a few inches in front of your nose. Do not stare, but keep your gaze relaxed and soft.

- Breathe naturally, allowing each breath to go in and out. Feel more relaxed with each breath.

- Release all thoughts from your mind. If a thought comes up, let it go like a passing cloud: it does not touch or affect you; it just passes by.

- In the beginning especially, you will likely have many thoughts that try to take over your mind. Do not get discouraged or judge yourself. Simply let each thought go and return to your breathing.

- When you are ready to stop, slowly raise your gaze and become aware of your surroundings.

- Meditate for about 10 of 15 minutes, twice a day if possible.

Walking Meditation

A variation of mindfulness meditation is walking meditation, a great way to combine meditation with a simple physical activity. If possible, choose a safe, tranquil place, such as a park, a quiet neighborhood, or even the track at a nearby high school or college.

Begin your walk by focusing on your breath. Allow your breathing to come naturally; do not try to control it in any way. Empty your mind of any thoughts and just stay with your breath. Once you have settled into focusing on your breath, shift your attention to your senses. Pay attention to your surroundings and experience them with your senses: listen to the birds; smell the air; feel the wind on your skin; notice the colors and shadows around you. Again, do not think. If thoughts creep into your head, let them go and return your attention to your breath or to your senses.

After a comfortable amount of time has passed, shift your attention to different parts of your body. As you walk, allow your attention to flow into your legs and feet. Notice how your feet feel as they touch the ground. Focus on the rhythm of your body and how each different part of your body moves as you walk. You may feel some warmth or tingling in each body part as you focus on it. Experience every sensation of your walk in a meditative, nonjudgmental way, as if you were a ray of light passing through the environment.

As you near the end of your walk, refocus on your breath and slowly return to your daily routine.

Progressive Muscle Relaxation

The practice of progressive muscle relaxation is one of the easiest and best ways to start and end your day, and you can do it while lying in bed. Progressive muscle relaxation can lower your blood pressure, reduce muscle tension, generate a sense of well-being, and improve blood flow to all parts of your body. If you do it before going to sleep, you'll never need to count sheep again!

You need only about fifteen minutes to do the full relaxation exercise. Don't rush through it, because that will defeat the purpose. The progression suggested here has been found to provide maximum relaxation:

- Find a quiet place where you can get into a comfortable position, lying down, sitting, or leaning back. You should not be wearing any restrictive clothing, such as shoes, belts, or tight pants.

- Breathe at a steady, slow pace throughout the exercise. Do not hold your breath or breathe faster.

- For each of the body parts mentioned, do the following: tense the muscles, hold the tension for five seconds, then relax the muscles gradually for 20 to 30 seconds as if you were letting air out of a balloon. As you release your tension, tell yourself that you are letting go, or visualize the stress draining from your body.

- **Chest.** Take a deep breath and send the air into your belly. Fill your lungs while you feel the tension in your chest. Exhale from the top of your lungs to your belly while you relax.

- **Left foot and lower leg.** Keep your heel down as you curl your toes back toward you until you feel the tension in your ankle and calf muscle.

- **Left upper leg.** Tense the top of your upper leg (quads) and the bottom of your upper leg (hamstring).

- **Right foot and lower leg.** Keep your heel down as you curl your toes back toward you until you feel the tension in your ankle and calf muscle.

- **Right upper leg.** Tense the top of your upper leg and the bottom of your lower leg.

- **Left hand and forearm.** Face your palm down as you lift your hand until you feel the tension in the top of the hand, the wrist, and the forearm.

- **Left upper arm.** Tense the biceps and triceps.

- **Left shoulder.** Shrug your left shoulder up toward your ear and roll your head toward your shoulder so your shoulder and ear are touching (if you can).

- **Right hand and forearm.** Face your palm down as you lift your hand until you feel the tension in the top of the hand, the wrist, and the forearm.

- **Right upper arm.** Tense the biceps and triceps.

- **Right shoulder.** Shrug your right shoulder up toward your ear and roll your head toward your shoulder so your shoulder and ear are touching (if you can).

- **Jaw.** Without damaging your teeth, bite down until you feel tension in your jaw.

- **Mouth.** Pretend you are whistling.

- **Chin.** Place the bottom of your tongue on the roof of your mouth and push upward.

- **Forehead.** Wrinkle your brow.

After you have practiced the progressive muscle relaxation technique regularly for several weeks, you should experience the full relaxation response. How will you recognize it? Your body will feel warm and heavy at first and then evolve into a feeling of weightlessness and complete relaxation.

Once you master this exercise, you will able to reach full relaxation in a shorter amount of time. Practice it often for a convenient and easy way to release your tension and stress.

Yoga

Yoga is a physical, mental, and spiritual discipline that has its roots in ancient India. The goal is to achieve tranquility and spiritual well-being, but you don't have to adhere to any spiritual or philosophical beliefs to practice yoga. In the United States, yoga is often used as a form of exercise and to relieve stress, and the specific discipline typically practiced is called hatha yoga. In fact, the three main features of hatha yoga—exercise, meditation, and breathing—make it an excellent choice for managing stress and stress-related illnesses, including heart disease, depression, asthma, insomnia, high blood pressure, anxiety, and pain.

Yoga and Aging

Yoga fights aging at a cellular level. Investigators at Ohio State University found that women who practiced yoga regularly had lower amounts of interleukin-6 (IL-6) in their blood. IL-6 is involved with inflammation and is associated with heart disease, stroke, type 2 diabetes, arthritis, and other age-related debilitating diseases. Ron Glaser, a coauthor of the study and a professor of molecular virology, immunology and medical genetics, explained that "yoga appears to be a simple and enjoyable way to add an intervention that might reduce risks for developing heart disease, diabetes and other age-related diseases." Experts at the Albert Einstein College of Medicine in New York have noted that practicing yoga may "promote restoration of physiologic setpoints to normal" after illness or injury and help restore balance at a cellular level.

Yoga: Getting Started

You don't need any fancy equipment to practice yoga—just comfortable clothing, no shoes, and a mat or thick, large towel for your floor postures. If you've never done yoga before, check with your doctor first, especially if you have any medical conditions. There are some yoga postures (usually the more advanced ones) that should be avoided if you have certain diseases.

It is helpful to learn the basics of yoga (hatha yoga is recommended for beginners) from a professional before you branch out on your own. You may find a class that offers free introductory sessions so you can discover whether you like it or not. Community centers, senior centers, hospitals, and clinics often offer yoga classes as well. Other sources of yoga instruction include videos and DVDs, which you can purchase or borrow from your local library; online instructions from a variety of Web sites, including YouTube; books; and TV.

Deep Breathing

What better way to defy aging than to master the very breath that keeps you alive! Even though you must breathe to live, most people don't practice true life-sustaining breathing. Proper breathing comes from the diaphragm—deep belly breathing—and not from the top of the chest, which is called shallow breathing. You should also breathe through your nose and not your mouth.

Take a moment and notice how you are breathing. Do your belly, lower back, and ribs expand when you take a breath? If not, then you are a shallow breather—and so are most people. But you can change that by practicing good breathing technique several times a day for just five to ten minutes. Here's how:

- Lie on your back or sit on the floor with your back against a wall so you are fully supported. Close your eyes and breathe normally for a minute.

- Practice breathing in and out of your nose only. Take slow, long breaths but not deep ones. Focus only on your breathing and how it feels. Do this for about 2 minutes.

- Now try to breathe with your belly. Put your hands on your stomach and see if they rise and fall as you breathe in and out. Concentrate on sending each breath down to your belly, but still don't breathe deeply, just slow and long. Practice for 2–3 minutes.

- Continue with the slow, long breaths and breathing into your belly, but now focus on your exhale. Make each exhale as long as each inhale. After a minute, try to make your exhales longer than your inhales. Practice this for a minute or two.

- You're done! Practice this exercise several times a day—while watching TV, when you first get up in the morning, before going to sleep at night, while riding public transportation, or while waiting in a long line.

Breathe Right, Live Longer

Breathing correctly can help you live longer, healthier, and smarter. If you don't believe it, here's why:

- **Breathing eliminates toxins.** Experts estimate that when you breathe properly, your body eliminates toxins and waste fifteen times faster than when you practice shallow breathing. Every time you exhale, you release carbon dioxide, a natural waste product of metabolism.

- **Breathing releases tension.** When you are stressed, your muscles become tense and your breathing is shallow. Proper breathing loosens up tight muscles and sends more oxygen to your cells.

- **Breathing improves brain function.** Proper breathing sends more oxygen to your brain cells, which can improve clarity, stimulate creativity, and raise awareness.

- **Breathing reduces pain.** People have a tendency to hold their breath when they anticipate or are experiencing pain. Holding your breath is counterproductive, because it can actually make the pain worse.

Breathing into your pain, however, offers some relief.

- **Breathing boosts the immune system.** When you maximize your breathing, you also enhance the amount of oxygen that binds to hemoglobin, which in turn enriches your body to metabolize nutrients and enhances immune system function.

- **Breathing strengthens muscles.** When you practice controlled breathing, it helps to strengthen and tone your abdominal muscles.

- **Breathing strengthens the lungs.** Dcep breathing can improve your lung function and help prevent respiratory problems.

- **Breathing improves heart function.** Breathing exercises benefit the heart by allowing it to not work as hard. Why? Because deep breathing makes your lungs work more efficiently, which sends more oxygen to the heart, which means the heart doesn't have to work as hard to deliver oxygen to the tissues throughout the body.

- **Breathing improves your mood.** Deep breathing increases production of neurochemicals in the brain responsible for pleasure, which in turn elevates your mood.

- **Breathing fights aging.** When you breathe in through your nose, the air flows over your pharynx, which is an area rich in nitric oxide. The flow of air allows the nitric oxide to enter the body, where it causes your arteries to open up and improves your circulation. Good circulation is necessary for healthy, young-looking skin, and a lack of nitric oxide can lead to premature aging.

Learn to Breathe Correctly

Have you ever watched infants breathe? They are belly breathers: their abdomens rise and fall with each inhalation. That's the way we are supposed to breathe: sending each breath deep into the abdomen, not just the chest. Here's how to breathe correctly. Schedule a minimum of five minutes twice a day to practice proper breathing techniques. Here's one for you to try:

- Keep your back straight while you do this exercise.

- Place the tip of your tongue against the back of your front teeth and keep it there while you do the breathing exercise.

- Exhale completely through your mouth, making a whoosh sound.

- Close your mouth and inhale through your nose. Send the air to your belly, then your chest, as you count to 4.

- Hold the breath for a count of 7.

- Exhale through your mouth to a count of 8.

- Repeat this cycle at least 3 more times.

You can do this breathing exercise just about anywhere: during a coffee break, while waiting in line, during your favorite TV show, or while preparing dinner. Whenever you begin to feel stressed, practice! This technique is also an excellent way to relax before going to sleep.

Tai Chi

Tai chi is a graceful form of exercise that originally developed in ancient China as a form of self-defense. Also known as tai chi chuan, the practice is often described as "meditation in motion" because it promotes calmness and tranquility through breathing and gentle movements that are performed in a slow, flowing manner. Although there are many different styles of tai chi, each with its own subtle methods and variations, they are all designed to achieve inner peace through coordinated breathing and movement.

Can practicing tai chi really reduce stress? Absolutely, and there is scientific evidence to support it. For example, one study looked at perceived stress, blood pressure, heart rate, and the level of cortisol (a stress hormone) in saliva in people who practiced tai chi for eighteen weeks. At the end of the study, the body told the story: saliva cortisol levels were significantly lower at the end of the study compared with the baseline values. Since cortisol levels are a good indicator of stress level, this reduction was an important indication that tai chi was effective in reducing stress. Mental stress was also significantly lower after the trial.

Researchers at Tufts University provide even more evidence. They reviewed forty studies that evaluated the psychological effects of tai chi. More than thirty-eight hundred people participated in the studies, most of which showed that the practice of tai chi significantly improved psychological well-being, including stress reduction, anxiety, and depression, and even improved self-esteem.

Getting Started

Most people find the best way to learn tai chi is in a class. Having an instructor will allow you to best experience the subtleties of the movements and breathing. Besides, performing tai chi with a group can be very liberating, like being part of a graceful dance group. Once you learn the basics, however, you can practice on your own or go on to learn new movements using DVDs or books for instructions. When performing tai chi, wear comfortable clothing that allows you to move and breathe freely. Shoes are optional and should be flat (e.g., ballet slippers).

Stress-Reducing Infusions (Teas)

A variety of herbal infusions/teas have stress-reducing qualities. Look for fresh dried forms of these herbs if available or, as an alternative, use tea bags. If you use the fresh dried herbs, steep the herb for ten minutes in water that has been boiled (remove water from heat once you add the herbs).

- **Black tea.** Even though it contains a small amount of caffeine, research shows that drinking black tea reduced levels of the stress hormone cortisol and helped make people feel calmer than individuals who drank a placebo with the same amount of caffeine.

- **Chamomile.** This is a longtime favorite herbal infusion to help relieve stress and help you sleep.

- **Ginseng.** Both Korean ginseng (*Panax schinsen*) and Siberian ginseng (*Eleutherococcus senticosus*) have properties that can boost resistance to stress. Perhaps even more important is that both types of ginseng are adaptogens, which means they have an ability to restore balance to the body. Use 1 teaspoon dried and chopped root per 8 ounces of water. Bring the water to a boil and simmer covered for fourteen to twenty minutes. Let stand until the tea is cool enough to drink.

- **Other favorite teas for stress.** Catnip, kava kava, passionflower, and skullcap.

Ten Easy, Fun Ways to Reduce Stress

- **Laugh.** When I get stressed from sitting at my computer for hours, I look for funny animal videos on the Internet. The Internet can be a rich source of humor—from funny videos to jokes, cartoons, movies, and humorous stories. Some people like to watch old reruns on TV (*I Love Lucy* always comes to mind) or DVDs of comedies or comedians. With today's high-tech cell phones, you can access a funny video just about any time you feel the pressure building up!

- **Soak.** A relaxing hot bath with aromatic oils can help melt away tension.

- **Dance to the music.** You don't need to go to a nightclub or party to dance: just turn up the music at home and let go. If you have a partner, great; if not, then improvise.

- **Listen to music.** What's your favorite—rock 'n' roll, classical, oldies, jazz? Turn it up, sing along, play air guitar, or conduct the orchestra.

- **Create something.** You don't need to be an artist to be creative. And no one even has to see what you make except you, but doing it can bring you a sense of peace. You might make a centerpiece or wreath using items you find in the park or woods. Try origami, painting a flowerpot, writing a poem, making a card for a friend . . . there are scores of things you can pour your stress into in a creative way.

- **Say no.** Sometimes you need to set boundaries and just say no. You can't please everyone all the time.

- **Enjoy a fragrance.** Some essential oils have been shown to have stress-reducing qualities. In fact, lavender is used in hospitals to calm patients. Also try oils of anise, basil, chamomile, eucalyptus, peppermint, rose, and thyme. Carry your aromatherapy with you: place a few pieces of rock salt in a small bottle or vial and add a few drops of your chosen oil. The rock salt will absorb the oil. Whenever you need a pick-me-up, take out the vial and enjoy the fragrance.

- **Write it down.** Sometimes simply putting your frustrations down on paper (or on a computer screen) can be a great stress reducer. Once your thoughts are in front of you, you can have a different perspective.

- **Cuddle an animal.** Petting and cuddling a dog or cat is a great way to bring down your blood pressure and relieve stress. If you don't have a pet of your own, visit a neighbor or friend who does. Volunteer to pet sit or walk their dog for them.

- **Be intimate.** If you have a partner, make a date to share some intimate time together. Have sex, give each other a massage, take a bubble bath together, read to each other—make it a time for both of you to let your stress go. Sex increases levels of mood-boosting chemicals in the brain called endorphins, a massage is a great tension reliever, and so is a hot bath.

STEP 10

Make Your Money Last

Do you dream of being financially secure after you retire? What if that desire is nothing more than a dream? Have you decided to put off retirement indefinitely because you can't afford it? The promise and dream of "financial security" has turned into a nightmare for many people, and especially for any who have lost their jobs, their homes, and some or all of their pension and other retirement monies. Economic changes that have erupted over the past several years have left adults of all ages, but especially middle-aged and older adults, facing new challenges concerning the integrity of their financial future. While attaining financial security can be a challenge, there is much you can do with careful planning to be secure.

The time to plan for your later years is now, even if you don't plan to retire. Yes, you may be among the increasing number of people who say they do not plan to retire at all or at least not until they are well into their seventies. That does not mean you don't need to create a financial plan, however. As part of your effort to add ten healthy years to your life, it's critical that you make efforts to ensure you have enough money to enjoy that extra decade as well as the years leading up to it! Having a firm, doable financial plan in place can help you feel more secure, and thus less anxious, and more able to manage the unexpected and to enjoy your life.

LATER-LIFE FINANCIAL CHALLENGES

The financial challenges you face in your later years will differ somewhat from those in your younger days, and they can present a significant burden if you don't figure them into your plan. One is the focus of this book: longer life. Over the years, average life expectancy has been slowly and gradually rising in the United States to nearly 80 years for women and 78 years for men. With effort on your part, you could extend those numbers by another decade or more, so you want to make sure you have sufficient income and assets for those years.

Along with living longer, other challenges associated with growing older can have a significant impact on your financial security and should be considered when you are planning your financial future.

- **Changes in your work and retirement.** Do you plan to continue working past the age of retirement? (See "Retire? Who, Me?") Will you need to work for the income, do you want to work because it provides mental stimulation and a sense of accomplishment—or is it a combination of both? If you plan to keep working well past traditional retirement age, you will need to consider what you do if you become physically and/or mentally unable to continue working as planned.

- **Caring for aging parents and parents-in-law.** You may be among the estimated 10 million adult children older than 50 who take care of their aging parents, according to a MetLife Mature Market Institute study released in 2011. The percentage of adults who provide personal and/or financial help for their parents has tripled since 1994, and the financial and emotional burdens on adult children can be enormous, especially if they need to interrupt or curtail their careers, which can jeopardize their own future financial security.

- **Changes in health.** Although many people have little problem remaining active and independent well into their later years, the possibility that health problems will develop, or that current ones will get more serious, must be faced. Thus it is important to pay for health insurance (beyond Medicare) and to consider how you will finance long-term care. About 80 percent of people older than 65 have at least one chronic health problem (e.g., arthritis, diabetes), and 50 percent have at least two. The better care you take of yourself starting right now, the better chance you have of living healthier and longer, but that still does not eliminate the need to plan for health care. Expect (and plan for) the unexpected!

- **Need for long-term care.** I hope you never need long-term health care, but if you do it can be extremely expensive. Most older people who need long-term care receive assistance from their spouses, children, and other family members. Providing this care can have a significant negative impact on the economic and emotional integrity of those providing the service, which is something you should consider whether you are on the giving or receiving end of this care. About 60 percent of people older than 65 will need some type of long-term care during their lifetime, and the average length of such care is three years. About 65 percent of people who need long-term care receive it entirely from family and friends.

- **Change in location.** You may decide you want or need to move out of your current housing arrangement. This can present either positive or negative effects on your financial situation, depending on the reasons for the move, as well as have an emotional impact on you.

- **Divorce.** Make sure you understand the laws regarding spousal rights to Social Security and retirement benefits if you get a divorce, especially if the divorce is late in life. You should also review your overall financial circumstances both before and after a divorce.

- **Death.** This is the change no one escapes. Preparing for your own death is an important task and includes funeral or burial planning as well as making sure your estate is in order with a will and estate planning. Be sure you have named your beneficiaries for any insurance policies, retirement plans, IRAs, and other retirement holdings.

RETIRE? WHO, ME?

A Wells Fargo survey of fifteen hundred Americans completed in November 2011 reported that 75 percent of middle-class Americans expect to work throughout the traditional retirement years (after age 65) and that 25 percent are so concerned about their savings, they plan to delay retirement until they are at least 80 years old. Given that life expectancy in the United States is 78 to 80 years, quite a few people plan to never retire. On the bright side, 42 percent of those surveyed said they would work at something that required "less responsibility."

Why are so many Americans pessimistic about their future? One reason is that, according to the survey, Americans have saved only 7 percent of the retirement stash they had hoped to accumulate. The average goal of people in the survey was $350,000, yet about 30 percent of people in their sixties said they had saved less than $25,000 for their retirement years.

Given the continuing poor economic climate in the United States—and much of the world for that matter—even $350,000 does not seem like it will last very long, especially if you face unexpected health challenges that may not be covered sufficiently or at all by Medicare, Medicaid, or insurance.

Getting Ready to Retire—at Any Age

The time to begin thinking about retirement is . . . now. If you're 25, 35, 45, and especially if you're even older, it's not enough to think about retirement—it's time to do something about it. Regardless of whether you are 25 and just starting your career path or 55 and looking forward to retirement, there are steps you should take to help ensure you will be financially secure in your older years.

The following suggestions can apply to adults of any age, but the older you are and the further away you are from your financial goals for retirement, the more aggressive you'll need to be to reach those goals. For example, let's say you are eligible for retirement in just a year or two, but the future looks uncertain because you (1) haven't saved enough money for a comfortable retirement or (2) lost a significant amount of your assets and now you don't have enough to retire on comfortably. Is it too late for you?

Absolutely not. The most important thing is to start immediately: it's only too late if you don't do anything right now! Warning: some of these suggestions may not be easy to swallow if you are late getting into financial planning for retirement, but they can make you feel more secure in the long run.

- **Evaluate your financial goals and be realistic.** Write them down; and if you have a partner, both of you should put your goals in writing. This gives you a starting point on which to focus. Your retirement vision may need to change, even dramatically. That will likely mean a less expensive lifestyle, but it doesn't have to mean an unhappy, less fulfilled one.

- **Define how much you need to save.** Break it down into a workable plan: is it $500 a month, $100 a week, $15 a day? Define a goal and stick with it. If possible, have the money earmarked for saving automatically deposited into a chosen account so you won't have to see it—but do monitor it so you know it is being deposited for you. For an eye-opening look at how much you may need to save, see the box "We Need How Much to Retire?"

- **Plan where to put your savings.** Look for places that provide the best tax advantages for you, such as a tax-sheltered retirement plan, tax-free bonds, an annuity. For help deciding how to best protect your savings, you need to educate yourself about the choices (go to the Appendix) and see if you can't get some free or low-cost professional advice.

- **Delay taking Social Security.** The longer you wait, the higher your monthly benefits will be.

- **Find ways to make extra money to reach your goal.** Here's where you may need to step outside your comfort zone and be creative and perhaps even ruthless. You might:
  - Take on extra work or a part-time job.
  - Sell any assets that are not producing income or that may become a liability in terms of maintenance or other factors in the near future. Examples include a vacation home, undeveloped land, jewelry, artwork, antiques, or other items of value that have not or likely will not appreciate any further.
  - Rent out a room in your home, space in your garage, or part of your land.
  - Downsize. Do you really need a big house and all the expenses that go along with it—energy costs, insurances, taxes, upkeep? Move to a less

expensive home and save any profits from the sale of your current residence. If you make such a move before you are forced into it, the transition will be a lot smoother and less stressful.

- Cut expenses. There are dozens of costs that can be reduced or eliminated; first you should list your regular and occasional expenses and then reevaluate each one. Some cuts may put you out of your comfort zone for a while, but if you approach the need for change as a chance to be creative it can take the sting out of it. (See "Cutting Expenses Without Bleeding.") Some cuts may yield only a few dollars per week or month, but when you add them up they can add up to a substantial amount of money for you to put away.

WE NEED HOW MUCH TO RETIRE?

According to Anthony Webb, an economist with the Center for Retirement Research at Boston College, a "typical" retired couple who are both 65 years old need the following amounts of savings to cover their out-of-pocket expenses for their remaining years (based on an average lifetime). These are estimates only, as Medicare, health-care costs, and other factors are constantly changing:

- For Medicare and other health premiums, drugs, copayments, and home health costs: $197,000.

- There is a 5 percent chance this amount could be as high as $311,000.

- If you include the possibility of nursing home costs, the original amount increases to $260,000.

- There is a 5 percent chance this amount could be greater than $517,000.

  A report from Fidelity Investments in 2011 offered a different perspective, but the figures are still high:

- A 65-year-old couple who retired in 2011 would need $230,000 to pay for medical care throughout their retirement years. This takes into account premiums, deductibles, and coinsurance associated with Medicare parts A, B, and D and some services not covered by Medicare. It does not include over-the-counter medications, most dental services, and long-term care and assumes women will live to age 85 and men to age 82.

CUTTING EXPENSES WITHOUT BLEEDING

If the thought of cutting expenses conjures up images of a slash-and-burn event that leaves your life in shambles, banish the thought. Often, cost-cutting measures reveal places where people have been wasting money needlessly, as in overpaying insurance premiums or for hidden services not used but paid for. Even if a few cost-cutting actions do hurt, time will heal your wounds and, with a little thought, you will discover ways to find alternatives to your slashed expenses, ways that may prove to be even better, healthier, and more fun than what you "lost".

- **Reevaluate your auto, home, renters', and other insurance policies.** Talk to your agent(s) about any cost-reducing steps you can take. Can you raise your deductibles? Is your car old enough so you can remove collision? Do you drive less? Has your home lost value, so that it now can be insured for a lower premium? Are you overinsured?

- **Reevaluate your phone bills.** Do you have both a landline and a cell phone? Do you really need both? Can you downgrade your cell phone plan or switch to a pay-as-you-go? Are you paying for services you don't really need?

- **Reevaluate your cable and/or Internet service.** Do you really need all the channels you pay for now? Can you significantly reduce or even eliminate your cable or satellite service? Can you bundle to save money?

- **Plan your driving trips to save gas.** When you have errands to run, write them down and plan to complete them as efficiently as possible.

- **Reevaluate your food shopping.** Are you buying brands and items that you can do without or that have a lower price substitute? Do you check the shopping flyers each week for specials? Do you use coupons? Do you shop at discount or dollar stores? Do stores in your area offer a senior-citizen discount day? You can realize significant savings if you take a little extra time to shop around and take advantage of specials, discount stores, and sales, switch to generic brands, and take up the challenge of preparing more low-cost healthy meals.

- **Reassess your entertainment and miscellaneous costs.** Movies, eating out, subscriptions, the daily latte, gifts: all of these can add up quickly and insidiously. If you're not aware of what you spend on these items, keep track for a few weeks or a month, then cut, cut, cut creatively. For example, there are free and low-cost entertainment options (e.g., borrow movies from the library, attend free lectures, look for free days at museums and galleries, take a hike, visit a park, join a book club or discussion group in your area or online). Find a free or low-cost option for the things you decide to change or cut. Need to give someone a gift? The gift of your time may be the most valued present he or she receives. Dare to think outside the box.

- **Cut energy costs.**
  - Lower your hot-water heater to 120 degrees Fahrenheit. Leaving the house for a week or longer? Turn the hot water dial to "vacation."
  - Lower your thermostat in the winter and dress warmer in the house
  - Seal any leaky doors, windows, and cracks.
  - Ask your utility company for a free energy audit.
  - Buying more energy-efficient appliances may be in order, but if you don't have the money to make a significant appliance purchase then you may need to find ways to make what you have more energy efficient. For example, use the cold/cold cycle on your washing machine, or hang your clothes out to dry instead of using the dryer. Keeping your refrigerator full (even if you put in bottles of water) uses less energy than if it is half-full, especially if you have an older model. To determine whether it is worth switching to a more energy-efficient appliance, including a heating and cooling system, do your homework. There are resources that can help you that are listed in the Appendix.

FINANCIAL LITERACY: WHAT DO YOU KNOW?

It's important that you identify your various sources of income and how you will manage them as retirement approaches or as you get older and your lifestyle and work habits change. For example, those sources may include a 401(k), IRAs, investments, annuities, employer-provided pensions, Social Security, rental income, or royalties. Managing these assets and various forms of income is different from receiving a regular paycheck, and juggling them can be complicated when income tax time rolls around as well.

So the important question is, How much do you know about your finances? One thing that is essential when making financial plans is to educate yourself about the basics—a Financial 101 per se. According to economist Joanne Hsu at the University of Michigan, financial literacy is low among both men and women in the United States. Hsu did research on how women prepare for the high likelihood their husbands would die first and leave them to handle the finances. Her sample showed that contrary to popular opinion, about 80 percent of the women were "on track" to reaching their husband's level of understanding about financial matters. If these women are left alone, they are likely to be successful at managing their money. That's the good news.

However, what if the husband's knowledge of or ability to handle the finances was not adequate? (I don't mean to be sexist here; there are certainly cases where the roles are reversed and the wife has managed the finances.) The point is, a little or inadequate knowledge of one's financial situation can be hazardous to his or her financial future. So, what should a couple do?

- The best scenario is for both partners in a marriage or other relationship where finances are shared to be fully aware of and involved in the financial decisions. Therefore, even if you are responsible for paying the bills and managing the banking, your partner should know what is going on, how much money you have, and where it is.

- A couple should plan for the likelihood that one of them will be left alone. The statistics bear this out: more than 75 percent of women who were previously married will become widows by the time they reach age 85. Women also tend to live an average of seventeen years after their husbands die. Sometimes a husband dies unexpectedly and the wife did not learn about their financial situation before his death. The worst time to take over finances is when you are in emotional turmoil and in an otherwise vulnerable situation in which others may take advantage of you. Therefore, plan for or get outside help to make sure there will be sufficient resources for the individual who is left behind.

Where to Get Financial Planning Help

If you have a financial adviser, he or she can help you with your questions. If you don't have a professional who can help you, reading books on basic financial and estate planning can be helpful (see Appendix), but it's usually best to find someone who can answer your questions one-on-one and explain nuances about different savings approaches. For affordable financial help, contact your local senior center, department of aging, and retirement centers to see if they offer any workshops, one-on-one counseling, or other financial help services. Check with your own bank or other financial institution where you do business to see what services they may offer you. You can also do the same with local banks and financial advisory firms with whom you do not do business.

Be careful when revealing your financial information. You are dealing with your life savings, your financial future—don't put it into the hands of just anyone. Do your homework! Check out any individual or firm you wish to help you with your finances. Don't think that just because a company has a well-known name you are safe. According to the Investment Adviser Association, a trade group, in 2005 an estimated 16 percent of registered investment advisory firms reported they had pending and past disciplinary proceedings ranging from violations of professional standards to breaking the law.

Now that your radar has been alerted, here are some tips from Consumer Reports' experts to help you avoid scams and incompetent advisers:

- **Look for an adviser who works for a fee, not on commission.** Preferably find a Certified Financial Planner (CFP). A Certified Financial Planner Board of Standards grants the CFP certification and has recognized standards of excellence for competent, ethical personal financial planning. The adviser should also have at least five years' experience.

- **Ask for the adviser's state registration.** Both independent advisers and companies paid to give out investment advice must register with the Securities and Exchange Commission (SEC).

- **Get Form ADV.** This form must be filed with the SEC by all registered financial advisers. Form ADV will tell you about any formal investment-related public disciplinary proceedings and legal judgments against the adviser, and it provides information on services, compensation, and potential conflicts of interest.

- **Check the Central Registration Depository.** This is a computerized database that lists information about most brokers, their representatives, and the firms they work for. You can get information about a broker's license, disciplinary record, work history, and educational history.

APPENDIX

ADVANCE DIRECTIVES

American Hospital Association
Offers an online brochure titled *Put it in Writing,* which provides basic facts about advance directives and helps individuals explore their preferences for end-of-life care.
http://www.putitinwriting.org/putitinwriting_app/index.jsp

Caring Connections
Download your state's advance directive forms free of charge.
http://www.caringinfo.org/i4a/pages/index.cfm?pageid=3289

Medline Plus
Many links to information about advance directives.
http://www.nlm.nih.gov/medlineplus/advancedirectives.html

DIET AND NUTRITION

American Institute for Cancer Research
Organization that funds cancer research and provides information for the public on how to help prevent and survive

a healthy diet, staying physically active,
ng a healthy weight.
.aicr.org/

Calorie Restriction Society International
The society's goal is to provide guidance for longer life and
better health based on continuing knowledge from different
branches of science concerning calorie restriction.
http://www.crsociety.org/

Center for Science in the Public Interest
Web site for a consumer advocacy organization that con-
ducts research and advocacy programs in nutrition and health
and provides consumers with information on same.
http://www.cspinet.org/

Consumer Lab
Reports on independent testing results of health and nutritional products.
http://www.consumerlab.com/

Mediterranean Diet
Information from the Mayo Clinic on the Mediterranean diet.
http://www.mayoclinic.com/health/mediterranean-diet/CL
00011

Okinawa Diet Online
This site follows the diet and lifestyle program from the
authors of *The Okinawa Program* and *The Okinawa Diet
Plan*.
http://okinawa-diet.com/

Preventive Medicine Research Institute
The Web site for Dr. Dean Ornish's organization, a nonprofit
research institute that performs scientific research investi-
gating the effects of diet and lifestyle choices on health
and disease.
http://www.pmri.org/

SAVINGS AND FINANCIAL PLANNING ASSISTANCE

Federal Trade Commission
How to protect yourself against identity theft.
http://www.ftc.gov/bcp/edu/microsites/idtheft/

LIFE Foundation
A nonprofit whose role is to educate the public about the essential role of life and health insurance in sound financial and retirement planning.
http://www.lifehappens.org/long-term-care-insurance
-introduction/

The Motley Fool
The Motley Fool is a multimedia financial services company that provides financial solutions for all types of investors, large and small, as well as financial information. The Motley Fool has products and services both online and offline, free and fee based, that are designed to help people take control of their finances.
http://www.fool.com/

MyFinancialAdvice.com
A Web site that offers some financial planning information and access to financial planners in your area (access by state), with an idea of what they charge for their services.
http://www.myfinancialadvice.com/Customer/Default
.aspx

U.S. Department of Energy
Energy Savers Booklet: *Tips on Saving Energy and Money at Home,* a thirty-six page booklet of tips on how to save energy in your home.
http://www.energysavers.gov/pdfs/energy_savers.pdf

U.S. Department of Labor

Savings Fitness: A Guide to Your Money and Your Financial Future, A comprehensive list of free publications
http://www.dol.gov/ebsa/publications/savingsfitness.html

A source of free e-books and booklets on personal finance, retirement, building wealth, and money management can be found at a website called mint.com
http://www.mint.com/blog/how-to/30-free-ebooks-to-learn -everything-you-want-to-know-about-personal-finance/

US Securities and Exchange Commission

Where to go to check out a brokerage firm, individual broker, individual investment adviser, or investment adviser firm.
http://www.sec.gov/answers/crd.htm

ENDNOTES

INTRODUCTION

T. Maruta et al. "Optimism-Pessimism Assessed in the 1960s and Self-Reported Health Status 30 Years Later," *Mayo Clin Proc* 77, no. 8 (August 2002): 748–53.

M. L. Kern et al., "Conscientiousness, Career Success, and Longevity: A Lifespan Analysis, *Ann Behav Med* 37, no. 2 (April 2009): 154–63.

STEP 1

"Position of the American Dietetic Association and Dietitians of Canada: Vegetarian Diets," *JADA* 103, no. 6 (2003): 748–65.

B. Aschebrooke-Kilfoy et al., "Epithelial Ovarian Cancer and Exposure to Dietary Nitrate and Nitrite in the NIH-AARP Diet and Health Study," *Eur J Cancer Prev,* September 20, 2011.

M. Collino, "High Dietary Fructose Intake: Sweet or Bitter Life?" *World J Diabetes* 2, no. 6 (June 15 2011): 77–81.

R. J. Johnson et al., "The Effect of Fructose on Renal Biology and Disease," *J Am SocNephrol* 21, no. 12 (December 2010): 2036–39.

M. Soffritti et al., "First Experimental Demonstration of the Multipotential Carcinogenic Effects of Aspartame Administered in the Feed to Sprague-Dawley rats," *Environ Health Perspect*; 114, no. 3 (March 2006): 379–85.

M. Soffritti et al., "Life-Span Exposure to Low Doses of Aspartame Beginning During Prenatal Life Increase Cancer Effects in Rats," *Environ Health Perspect* 115, no. 9 (September 2007): 1293–97.

J. Uribarri et al., "Circulating Glycotoxins and Dietary Advanced Glycation End Products: Two Links to Inflammatory Response, Oxidative Stress, and Aging," *J Gerontol A BiolSci Med Sci* 62, no. 4 (April 2007): 427–33.

STEP 2

A. M. Egras et al., "An Evidence-Based Review of Fat Modifying Supplemental Weight Loss Products," *J Obesity,* 2011, p. ii: 297315.

A.M. Valdes et al., "Obesity, Cigarette Smoking, and Telomere Length in Women," *Lancet* 366, no. 9486 (August 20–26, 2005): 662–64.

STEP 3

R. Andel et al., "Physical Exercise at Midlife and Risk of Dementia Three Decades Later," *J Gerontol A BiolSci Med Sci* 63, no. 1 (June 2008): 62–66.

J. L. Steiner et al., "Exercise Training Increases Mitochondrial Biogenesis in the Brain," *J Appl Physiol,* August 4, 2011. 111(4): 1066–71.

H. Van Praag, "Neurogenesis and Exercise: Past and Future Directions," *Neuromolecular Med,* February 20, 2008.

J. L. Veerman et al., "Television Viewing Time and Reduced Life Expectancy: A Life Table Analysis," *Br J Sports Med* August 15, 2011, online.

C. P. Wen et al., "Minimum Amount of Physical Activity for Reduced Mortality and Extended Life Expectancy: A Prospective Cohort Study," *Lancet,* August 16, 2011.

C. W. Wu et al., "Treadmill Exercise Counteracts the Suppressive Effects of Peripheral Lipopolysaccharide on Hippocampal Neurogenesis and Learning and Memory," *J Neurochem* 103, no. 6 (December 2007): 2471–81.

STEP 4

"Pneumonia Vaccine," Medscape, http://www.medscape .com/viewarticle/753734.

American Health Information Management Association (AHIMA), http://www.myphr.com/Default.aspx.

Federal Trade Commission, "Tips on How to Avoid Identify Theft," www.ftc.gov/idtheft.

STEP 5

R. Andel et al., "Physical Exercise at Midlife and Risk of Dementia Three Decades Later," *J Gerontol A BiolSci Med Sci* 63, no. 1 (January 2008): 62–66.

M. Assuncao et al., "Red Wine Antioxidants Protect Hippocampal Neurons Against Ethanol-Induced Damage," *Neuroscience* 146, no. 4 (June 8, 2007): 1581–92.

S. S. Bassuk et al., "Social Disengagement and Incident Cognitive Decline in Community-Dwelling Elderly Persons," *Ann Intern Med* 131, no. 3 (August 3, 1999): 165–73.

S. Bastianetto et al., "Neuroprotective Abilities of Resveratrol and Other Red Wine Constituents Against Nitric Oxide-Related Toxicity in Cultured Hippocampal Neurons," *Br J Pharmacol* 131, no. 4 (October 2000): 711–20.

Y. Chen et al., "Rapid Loss of Dendritic Spines After Stress Involves Derangement of Spine Dynamics by Corticotrophin-Releasing Hormone," *J Neurosci* 28, no. 11 (March 12, 2008): 2903–11.

S. Gais and J. Born, "Declarative Memory Consolidation: Mechanisms Acting During Human Sleep," *Learn Mem* 11, no. 6 (November—December 2004): 679–85.

R. L. Galli et al., "Blueberry Supplemented Diet Reverses Age-Related Decline in Hippocampal HSP70 Neuroprotection," *Neurobiol Aging* 27, no. 2 (February 2006): 344–50.

R. Guzman-Marin et al., "Rapid Eye Movement Sleep Deprivation Contributes to Reduction of Neurogenesis in the Hippocampal Dentate Gyrus of the Adult Rat," *Sleep* 31, no. 2 (February 1, 2008): 167–75.

L. O. Kurlak and T.J. Stephenson, "Plausible Explanations for Effects of Long Chain Polyunsaturated Fatty Acids (LCPUFAs) on Neonates," *Arch Dis Child Fetal Neonatal Ed* 80, no. 20 (March 1999): 148–54.

H. Lau et al., "Daytime Napping: Effects on Human Direct

Associative and Relational Memory," *Neurobiol Learn Mem* 93, no. 4 (May 2010): 554–60.

S. J. Lupien et al., "Stress Hormones and Human Memory Function Across the Lifespan," *Psychoneuroendocrinology* 30, no. 3 (April 2005): 225–42.

J. L. Madrigal et al., "Stress-Induced Oxidative Changes in Brain," *CNS NeurolDisord* 5, no. 5 (October 2006): 561–68.

M. C. Morris et al., "Associations of Vegetable and Fruit Consumption with Age-Related Cognitive Change," *Neurology* 67, no. 8 (October 24, 2008): 1370–76.

G. Ravaglia et al., "Homocysteine and Folate as Risk Factors for Dementia and Alzheimer Disease," *Am J ClinNutr* 82, no. 3 (September 2005): 636–43.

S. R. Schmidt, "Effects of Humor on Sentence Memory," *J Exp Psychol Learn MemCogn* 20, no. 4 (July 1994): 953–67.

M. A. Tucker and W. Fishbein, "Enhancement of Declarative Memory Performance Following a Daytime Nap Is Contingent on Strength of Initial Task Acquisition," *Sleep* 31, no. 2 (February 1, 2008): 197–203.

J. Verghese et al., "Leisure Activities and the Risk of Dementia in the Elderly," *N Engl J Med* 348, no. 25 (June 19, 2003): 2508–16.

U. Wagner and J. Born, "Memory Consolidation During Sleep: Interactive Effects of Sleep Stages and HPA Regulation," *Stress* 20 (July 2007): 1.

C. W. Wu et al., "Treadmill Exercise Counteracts the Suppressive Effects of Peripheral Lipopolysaccharide on Hippocampal Neurogenesis and Learning and Memory," *J Neurochem* 103, no. 6 (December 2007): 2471–81.

H. Van Praag, "Neurogenesis and Exercise: Past and Future Directions," *Neuromolecular Med,* February 20, 2008. 8680–85.

M. A. Yoder and R.H. Haude, "Sense of Humor and Longevity: Older Adults' Self-Ratings Compared with Ratings for Deceased Siblings," *Psychol Rep* 76, no. 3, part 1 (June 1995): 945–46.

O. Ybarra et al., "Social Interaction Promotes General Cognitive Functioning," *Pers Soc Psychol Bull* 34, no. 2 (February 2008): 248–59.

STEP 6

"Pterostilbene's Healthy Potential," *Agricultural Research,* November—December 2006 online.

J. A. Alosi et al., "Pterostilbene Inhibits Breast Cancer in Vitro Through Mitochondrial Depolarization and Induction of Caspase-Dependent Apoptosis," *J Surg Res* 161, no. 2 (June 15, 2010): 195–201.

M. Amarnath Satheesh and L. Pari, "The Antioxidant Role of Pterostilbene in Streptozotocin-Nicotinamide-Induced Type 2 Diabetes Mellitus in Wistar Rats," *J Pharm Pharmacol* 58, no. 11 (November 2006): 1483–90.

H. Ansar et al., "Effects of Alpha-Lipoic Acid on Blood Glucose, Insulin Resistance and Glutathione Peroxidase of Type 2 Diabetic Patients," *Saudi Med J* 32, no. 6 (June 2011): 584–88.

J. L. Barger et al., "A Low Dose of Dietary Resveratrol Partially Mimics Caloric Restriction and Retards Aging Parameters in Mice," *PLoS One* 3, no. 6 (2008): e2264.

D. J. Boocock et al., "Phase I Dose Escalation Pharmacokinetic Study in Healthy Volunteers of Resveratrol, a Potential Cancer Chemopreventive Agent," *Cancer Epidemiol Biomarkers Prev* 16, no. 6 (2007): 1246–52.

J. Chang et al., "Low-Dose Pterostilbene, but Not Resveratrol, Is a Potent Neuromodulator in Aging and Alzheimer's Disease," *Neurobiol Aging,* October 2011 online.

Y. S. Chiou et al., "Pterostilbene Inhibits Colorectal Aberrant Crypt Foci (ACF) and Colon Carcinogenesis Via Suppression of Multiple Signal Transduction Pathways in Azoxymethane-Treated Mice," *J Agric Food Chem* 58, no. 15 (August 11, 2010): 8833–41.

Y. S. Chiou et al., "Pterostilbene Is More Potent than Resveratrol in Preventing Azoxymethane (AOM)–Induced Colon Tumorigenesis via Activation of the NF-E2-Related Factor 2 (Nrf2)-Mediated Antioxidant Signaling Pathway," *J Agric Food Chem* 59, no. 6 (March 23, 2011): 2725–33.

M. Chung et al., *Vitamin D and Calcium: Systematic Review of Health Outcomes,* Evidence Report/Technology Assessment No. 183 (prepared by Tufts Evidence-based Practice Center under Contract No. 290-2007-10055-I), AHRQ Publication No. 09-E015 (Rockville, MD: Agency for Healthcare Research and Quality, August 2009).

D. K. Das et al., "Resveratrol and Red Wine, Healthy Heart and Longevity," *Heart Fail Rev* 15, no. 5 (September 2010): 467–77.

S. Dixit et al., "Protective Role of Exogenous Alpha-Lipoic Acid (ALA) on Hippocampal Antioxidant Status and Memory Function in Rat Pups Exposed to Sodium Arsenite During the Early Post-natal Period," *Toxicol Mech Methods* 21, no. 3 (March 2011): 216–24.

E. K. Farina et al., "Protective Effects of Fish Intake and Interactive Effects of Long-Chain Polyunsaturated Fatty Acid Intakes on Hip Bone Mineral Density in Older Adults: The Framingham Osteoporosis Study," *Am J ClinNutr* 93, no. 5 (May 2011): 1142–51.

A. Faust et al., "Effect of Lipoic Acid on Cyclophosphamide-Induced Diabetes and Insulitis in Non-obese Diabetic Mice," *Int J Immunopharmacol* 16 (1994): 61–66.

G. Fernandes et al., "Effects of N-3 Fatty Acids on Autoimmunity and Osteoporosis," *Front Biosci* 13 (May 1, 2008): 4015–20.

"Glutathione Information," http://www.themaxsite.com/benefits.html.

E. K. Go et al., "Betaine Suppresses Proinflammatory Signaling During Aging: The Involvement of Nuclear Factor Kappa B via Nuclear Factor–Inducing Kinase/IkappaB Kinase and Mitogen-Activated Protein Kinases," *J Gerontol Biol Sci* 60A, no. 10 (2005): 1252–64.

N. Harada et al., "Resveratrol Improves Cognitive Function in Mice by Increasing Production of Insulin-like Growth Factor-I in the Hippocampus," *J NutrBiochem* 22, no. 12 (2011): 1150–59.

M. Hashimoto and S. Hossain, "Neuroprotective and Ameliorative Actions of Polyunsaturated Fatty Acids Against Neuronal Diseases: Beneficial Effect of Docosahexaenoic Acid on Cognitive Decline in Alzheimer's Disease," *J PharmacolSci* 116, no. 2 (2011): 150–62.

K. A. Head, "Natural Therapies for Ocular Disorders, Part Two: Cataracts and Glaucoma," *Altern Med Rev* 6, no. 2 (2001): 141–66.

J. E. Joseph et al., "Cellular and Behavioral Effects of Stilbene Resveratrol Analogues: Implications for Reducing the Deleterious Effects of Aging," *J Agric Food Chem* 56 (2008): 10544–51.

Julius M. et al., Glutathione and Morbidity in a Community-based Sample of Elderly. *J Clin Epidemiol* 1994 Sept; 47(9): 1021–26

J. P. Kesby et al., "The Effects of Vitamin D on Brain Development and Adult Brain Function," *Mol Cell Endocrinol* 347, no. 1–2 (December 5, 2011): 121–27.

L. Li et al., "Vascular Oxidative Stress and Inflammation Increase with Age: Ameliorating Effects of Alpha-Lipoic Acid Supplementation," *Ann NY AcadSci* 1203 (August 2010): 151–59.

"Linus Pauling Institute," http://lpi.oregonstate.edu/infocenter/othernuts/coq10/.

D. J. Llewellyn et al., "Vitamin D and Cognitive Impairment in the Elderly US Population," *J Gerontol A Biol Sci Med Sci* 66, no. 1 (January 2011): 59–65.

L. Lv et al., "Stilbeneglucoside from Polygonum Multiflorumthunb: A Novel Natural Inhibitor of Advanced Glycation End Product Formation by Trapping of Methylglyoxal," *J Agric Food Chem* 58, no. 4 (February 24, 2010): 2239–45.

D. J. McKenna et al., "Green Tea Monograph," *Alt Ther* 6, no. 3 (2000): 61–84.

P. W. Mannal et al., "Pterostilbene Inhibits Pancreatic Cancer in Vitro," *J GastrointestSurg* 14, no. 5 (May 2010): 873–79.

B. Merle et al., "Dietary Omega-3 Fatty Acids and the Risk for Age-Related Maculopathy: The Alienor Study," *Invest Ophthalmol Vis Sci* 52, no. 8 (July 29, 2011): 6004–11.

M. F. Melhem et al., "Effects of Dietary Supplementation of Alpha-Lipoic Acid on Early Glomerular Injury in Diabetes Mellitus," *J Am Soc Nephrol* no. 12 (2001): 124–33.

Y. Miura et al., "Tea Catechins Prevent the Development of Atherosclerosis in Apoprotein E-Deficient Mice," *J Nutr* 131, no. 1 (2001): 27–32.

D. Moran, "Calcium's Effect on Brain Functions," *Natural Products Marketplace,* April 10, 2007: 40.

D. Mozaffarian and J. H. Wu, "Omega-3 Fatty Acids and Cardiovascular Disease: Effects on Risk Factors, Molecular Pathways and Clinical Events," *J Am CollCardiol* 58, no. 20 (November 8, 2011): 2047–67.

T. Nagao et al., "A Green Tea Extract High in Catechins Reduces Body Fat and Cardiovascular Risks in Humans," *Obesity* (Silver Spring) 15, no. 6 (2007): 1473–83.

Office of Dietary Supplements, National Institutes of Health, http://ods.od.nih.gov/factsheets/calcium.

M.H. Pan et al., "Pterostilbene Inhibited Tumor Invasion via Suppressing Multiple Signal Transduction Pathways in Human Hepatocellular Carcinoma Cells," *Pterostilbene Inhibits Liver Cancer*, no. 7 (July 2009): 1234–42.

E.S. Park et al., "Pterostilbene, a Natural Dimethylated Analog of Resveratrol, Inhibits Rat Aortic Vascular Smooth Muscle Cell Proliferation by Blocking Akt-Dependent Pathway," *Vascul Pharmacol* 53, no. 1–2 (July 2010): 61–67.

"Pterostilbene Monograph," *Altern Med Rev* 15, no. 2 (2010): 159–63.

J. L. Quiles et al., "Life-long Supplementation with a Low Dosage of Coenzyme Q10 in the Rat: Effects on Antioxidant Status and DNA Damage," *Biofactors* 25, no. 1–4 (2005): 73–86.

A. C. Ross et al., *Dietary Reference Intakes for Calcium and Vitamin D* (National Academies Press, Washington, DC, 2011).

J. G. Schneider et al., "Pterostilbene Inhibits Lung Cancer Through Induction of Apoptosis," *J Surg Res* 161, no. 1 (June 1, 2010): 18–22.

R. Sheng et al., "Epigallocatechingallate, the Major Component of Polyphenols in Green Tea, Inhibits Telomere Attrition Mediated Cardiomyocyte Apoptosis in Cardiac Hypertrophy," *Int J Cardiol,* October 14, 2011.

A. D. Smith et al., "Homocysteine-Lowering by B Vitamins Slows the Rate of Accelerated Brain Atrophy in Mild Cognitive Impairment: A Randomized Controlled Trial," *PLoS ONE* 5, no. 9 (2010): e12244.

A. Steptoe et al., "The Effects of Chronic Tea Intake on Platelet Activation and Inflammation: A Double-Blind Placebo Controlled Trial," *Atherosclerosis* 193, no. 2 (2007): 277–82.

University of Maryland Medical Center, http://www.umm .edu/altmed/articles/coenzyme-q10-000295.htm.

J. L. Vacekk et al., "Vitamin D Deficiency and Supplementation and Relation to Cardiovascular Health," *Am J Cardiol,* November 7, 2011.

T. J. Wang et al., "Vitamin D Deficiency and Risk of Cardio-vascular Disease," *Circulation* 117, no. 4 (January 29, 2008): 503–11.

B. M. Wolpin et al., "Plasma 25-Hydroxyvitamin D and Risk of Pancreatic Cancer," *Cancer Epidemiol Biomarkers Prev,* November 15, 2011.

STEP 7

S. S. Bassuk et al., "Social Disengagement and Incident Cognitive Decline in Community-Dwelling Elderly Persons," *Ann Intern Med* 131, no. 3 (August 3, 1999): 165–73.

M. G. Berman et al., "The Cognitive Benefits of Interacting with Nature," *Psychol Science* 19, no. 12 (December 2008): 1207–12.

R. Berto, "Exposure to Restorative Environments Helps Restore Attentional Capacity," *J Environ Psych* 25, no. 3 (September 2005): 249–59.

J. Holt-Lunstad et al., "Influence of a 'Warm Touch' Support Enhancement Intervention Among Married Couples on Ambulatory Blood Pressure, Oxytocin, Alpha Amylase, and Cortisol," *Psychosom Med* 70, no. 9 (November 2008): 976–85.

B. H. Gottlieb and A.A. Gillespie, "Volunteerism, Health, and Civic Engagement Among Older Adults," *Can J Aging* 27, no. 4 (Winter 2008): 399–406.

N. Morrow-Howell, "Volunteering in Later Life: Research Frontiers," *J Gerontol B Psychol Sci Soc Sci* 65, no. 4 (July 2010): 461–69.

F. Kuo and the National Recreation and Park Association, *Parks and Other Green Environments: Essential Compo-*

nents of a Healthy Human Habitat: Executive Summary, National Recreation and Park Association, 2010.

J. Maas et al., "Morbidity Is Related to a Green Living Environment," *J Epidemiol Comm Health* 63 (2009): 967–73.

James W. Pennebaker Ph.D., *Opening Up: The Healing Power of Confiding in Others.* (New York: William Morrow, 1990), pp. 118–19.

Benedict Carey, "Evidence That Little Touches Do Mean So Much," *New York Times,* February 22, 2010, http://www.nytimes.com/2010/02/23/health/23mind.html.

O. Ybarra et al., "Social Interaction Promotes General Cognitive Functioning," *PersSocPsychol Bull* 34, no. 2 (February 2008): 248–59.

Good Morning America, http://abcnews.go.com/GMA/On-Call/Story?id=7037716&page=1.

STEP 8

L. Abenavoli et al., "Milk Thistle in Liver Diseases: Past, Present, Future," *Phytother Res* 24, no. 10 (October 2010): 1423–32.

http://www.vrp.com/liver-support/healthy-aging-protection-against-common-environmental-toxins.

E. Kandaraki et al., "Endocrine Disruptors and Polycystic Ovary Syndrome (PCOS): Elevated Serum Levels of Bisphenol A in Women with PCOS," *J ClinEndocrinolMetab* 96, no. 3 (March 2011): E480–84.

David Perlmutter M. D. FACN, *The Better Brain Book* (Riverhead, New York, 2004).

A. Shankar and S. Teppala, "Relationship Between Urinary Bisphenol A Levels and Diabetes Mellitus," *J Clin-EndocrinolMetab,* September 28, 2011.

A. S. Tomlin et al., "A Field Study of Factors Influencing the Concentrations of a Traffic-Related Pollutant in the Vicinity of a Complex Urban Junction," *Atmospheric Environment* 43, no. 32 (October 2006): 5027–37.

STEP 9

T. Esch et al., "Mind/Body Techniques for Physiological and Psychological Stress Reduction: Stress Management via Tai Chi Training—a Pilot Study," *Med SciMonit* 13, no. 11 (November 2007): cr488–97.

Disabled World, "Yoga Reduces Inflammation Due to Aging and Stress." http://www.disabled-world.com/fitness/exercise/yoga/yoga-inflammation-stress.php#ixzz1ZU0Cpe3E.

E. Epel et al., "Can Meditation Slow Rate of Cellular Aging? Cognitive Stress, Mindfulness, and Telomeres," *Ann NY Acad Sci* 1172 (August 2009): 34–53.

J. K. Iecolt-Glaser et al., "Stress, Inflammation, and Yoga Practice," *Psychosom Med* 72, no. 2 (February 2010): 113–21.

Thich Nhat Hanh recommends it strongly in his book on walking meditation, *The Long Road Turns to Joy.* Berkeley, CA: Parallax Press, 1996.

V. Kuntsevich et al., "Mechanisms of Yogic Practices in Health, Aging, and Disease," *Mt Sinai J Med* 77, no. 5 (September–October 2010): 559–69.

B. A. Shaw et al., "Are Changes in Financial Strain Associated with Changes in Alcohol Use and Smoking Among

Older Adults?" *J Studies Alcohol Drugs* 72, no. 6 (November 2011): 917–25.

E. S. Epel et al., "Accelerated Telomere Shortening in Response to Life Stress," *Proceedings of the National Academy of Science USA* 101, no. 49 (December 7, 2004): 17312–25.

M. Wikgren et al., "Short Telomeres in Depression and the General Population Are Associated with a Hypocortisolemic State," *Biological Psychiatry,* November 2011.

Jen Weigel, "Stress and Aging: Slow It Down," *Chicago Tribune,* September 15, 2010, http://articles.chicagotribune.com/2010-09-15/features/ct-tribu-weigel-stress-20100915_1_elissa-epel-stress-cells-age.

C. Wang et al., "Tai Chi on Psychological Well-Being: Systematic Review and Meta-analysis," *BMC Complement Altern Med* 10 (May 21, 2010): 23.

STEP 10

"MetLife Study of Caregiving Costs to Working Caregivers: Double Jeopardy for Baby Boomers Caring for Their Parents," http://www.metlife.com/about/press-room/index.html?compID=49334, accessed December 3, 2011.

Wells Fargo survey, http://finance.yahoo.com/news/25-americans-expect-wait-until-181500675.html.

Financial Security Project at Boston College, http://fsp.bc.edu/tag/aging/.

Fidelity Investments report, http://money.usnews.com/money/blogs/planning-to-retire/2011/03/31/fidelity-couples-need-230000-for-retirement-health-costs, accessed December 3, 2011.

SUGGESTED READING

Chopra, Sanjiv, and Alan Lotvin. *Doctor Chopra Says: Medical Facts & Myths Everyone Should Know.* New York: St. Martin's Press, 2010.

Delaney, Brian M., and Lisa Walford. *The Longevity Diet: Discover Calorie Restriction—the Only Proven Way to Slow the Aging Process and Maintain Peak Vitality.* Cambridge, MA: Da Capo Press, 2005.

Garavaglia, Jan. *How Not to Die: Surprising Lessons on Living Longer, Safer, and Healthier.* New York: Crown Publishers, 2008.

Hallisy, Julia A. *The Empowered Patient.* San Francisco: PatientsafetyCA.org, 2008.

Kushner, Thomasine. *Surviving Health Care: A Manual for Patients and Their Families.* Cambridge: Cambridge University Press, 2010.

Liponis, Mark. *Ultralongevity: The Seven-Step Program for a Younger, Healthier You.* New York: Little, Brown, 2007.

Ornish, Dean. *Dr. Dean Ornish's Program for Reversing Heart Disease: The Only System Scientifically Proven to Reverse Heart Disease Without Drugs or Surgery.* New York: Ivy Books, 1995.

———. *Love & Survival: The Scientific Basis for the Healing Power of Intimacy.* New York: HarperCollins, 1997.

———. *The Spectrum: A Scientifically Proven Program to*

Feel Better, Live Longer, Lose Weight, and Gain Health. New York: Ballantine, 2008.

Pennebaker, James W. Ph.D. *Opening Up: The Healing Power of Confiding in Others.* New York: William Morrow, 1990.

Walford, Roy L., and Lisa Walford. *The Anti-Aging Plan: The Nutrient-Rich, Low-Calorie Way of Eating for a Longer Life—the Only Diet Scientifically Proven to Extend Your Healthy Years.* Cambridge, MA: Da Capo Press, 2005.

Weil, Andrew. *Spontaneous Happiness.* New York: Little, Brown, 2011.